Understanding Clinical Cardiac Electrophysiology

Understanding Clinical Cardiac Electrophysiology

A Conceptually Guided Approach

Peter Spector, MD

Professor of Medicine,
Director, Cardiac Electrophysiology and Cardiac Electrophysiology Laboratory,
University of Vermont Medical Center,
University of Vermont College of Medicine
Burlington, VT, USA

WILEY Blackwell

Published by John Wiley & Sons, Inc., Hoboken, New Jersey
Published simultaneously in Canada

For general information on our other products and services or for technical support, please contact our Customer Care Department within the United States at (800) 762-2974, outside the United States at (317) 572-3993 or fax (317) 572-4002.

Wiley also publishes its books in a variety of electronic formats. Some content that appears in print may not be available in electronic formats. For more information about Wiley products, visit our web site at www.wiley.com.

Library of Congress Cataloging-in-Publication Data:

Names: Spector, Peter, author.
Title: Understanding clinical cardiac electrophysiology : a conceptually guided approach / Peter Spector.
Description: Chichester, West Sussex, UK ; Hoboken, NJ : John Wiley & Sons Inc., 2016. |
    Includes bibliographical references and index.
Identifiers: LCCN 2015043776 | ISBN 9781118905494 (paperback)
Subjects: | MESH: Electrophysiologic Techniques, Cardiac. | Arrhythmias, Cardiac. |
    Atrial Function. | Cardiac Electrophysiology–methods.
Classification: LCC RC683.5.E5 | NLM WG 141.5.F9 | DDC 616.1/207547–dc23
LC record available at http://lccn.loc.gov/2015043776

Set in 10.5/13.5pt Minion by SPi Global, Pondicherry, India
Printed and bound in Singapore by Markono Print Media Pte Ltd

10 9 8 7 6 5 4 3 2 1

1 2016

Contents

Preface

Why this book?

I don't know about you, but my shelves are brimming with texts on cardiac electrophysiology. EP texts range from colossal reference tomes to "tips and tricks." Despite all of the material available to students and practitioners, I was inspired to write this book by the perception of a void. In the fast-paced world of clinical training students are often inundated with the "what" of electrophysiology without the "why." *Understanding Clinical Cardiac Electrophysiology* is designed to tell the story of electrophysiology so that the seemingly disparate myriad observations of clinical practice come into focus as a cohesive and predictable whole. While it can be difficult to memorize a thousand words, it is easy to remember a single story.

Cardiac electrophysiology as a "complex non-linear system"

Science has undergone a revolution of sorts in the past 60 years. Despite its incredible accomplishments, science had been relatively ill equipped to address the behavior of systems composed of multiple interdependent parts. An emerging discipline has focused on understanding how such systems change over time. "Systems" as diverse as the economy, the brain, and army ants are all "complex non-linear dynamic systems." The meaning of this unfamiliar and somewhat daunting phrase is captured by the expression "the whole is greater than the sum of its parts." Even with an understanding of how individual elements of such a system "work," and of the "rules of engagement" that govern their interactions, it can be difficult or impossible to predict the behavior of complex non-linear systems more than a short time into the future. There is often no *analytic* solution to predict the behavior of complex systems – i.e., there is no formula that converts starting values into future values at arbitrarily distant times. Often the only way to determine behavior is to iteratively calculate how each new state of the system evolves into the next state. This process of iterative assessment is tremendously aided by modern computers. Whereas humans may be able to mentally compute a few steps, they quickly fatigue and "lose track." Computers never fatigue and are now capable of computing at such blinding speeds that they can quickly demonstrate the evolution of systems through time.

I had been studying cardiac electrophysiology for many years but was entirely unaware of the existence of complex systems or the notion of emergent behavior. When I was introduced to these ideas by a colleague[1] it became clear that cardiac electrophysiology is a classic example of a complex non-linear dynamic system, and that the science of such systems can offer many insights germane to understanding electrophysiology. Over the six years leading up to the writing of this book I began meeting with some particularly intelligent and curious colleagues and students to discuss electrophysiology and how it can best be understood. These discussions evolved into a weekly meeting of faculty and fellows dubbed "the EP study group." These meetings had a loose and wide-ranging agenda; the EP study group was more of an ongoing conversation than a lecture. We began with the question: "What are we really measuring when we record electrograms?" This led to a six-year-long journey that included a review of vector calculus, Maxwell's equations, discussions of neural networks and other forms of artificial intelligence, complexity, genetic algorithms, and on and on. This book has in part been an attempt to codify the lessons learned and present them to a wider audience. Fear not, this is not a book about the heart as a complex system; but it does tell its story informed by this powerful perspective.

---

[1] Jason H. T. Bates PhD, DSc

"The heart is a computer"

I have come to appreciate that the heart isn't "like" a computer; in a very meaningful way it *is* a computer. It is an enormous parallel processor. Based upon the rules that govern the behavior of individual cells, the interactions between cells, and the structure which connects these cells, the heart begins with its current "state" and calculates its next state. From this perspective one can appropriately say "your heart is a computer; your rhythm is the result of its ongoing calculation."

Despite the fact that the material and perspective described above is unfamiliar to most clinical electrophysiologists, this book is very much written for clinicians. These ideas are harnessed in order to facilitate a deeper understanding of electrophysiology, both to appreciate its infinite aesthetic beauty and *in order that such understanding may be used to practice better electrophysiology.*

The proper treatment of cardiac electrophysiology requires some mathematics, particularly when it comes to the physics of excitable tissue and the development of computational models. Such mathematics, which is essential for a proper understanding of the subject, is often eschewed by physiologists and medical practitioners and left to the biophysicist and biomedical engineer. One of my goals in the present book is to bridge this culture gap by making the necessary mathematics as accessible as possible to those who might not normally consider themselves that way inclined (I am one such person). Because some respond to mathematics with either panic or coma, I have placed the mathematics in an appendix where it can safely be ignored by those so inclined.

What this book isn't

Understanding Clinical Cardiac Electrophysiology is not a textbook of electrophysiology. It is not a manual of operations for procedures. It does not focus on specific diagnostic criteria. It does not address implementation of therapeutic interventions. Numerous other sources are available for addressing these important aspects of cardiac electrophysiology. If you are going to read only one book about electrophysiology ... don't read this one. My objective is to review the principles that underlie electrophysiology and the analytic tools which, when combined with a firm grasp of EP mechanisms, allow readers to think through any situation in which they find themselves.

Acknowledgments

My first deep exposure to electrophysiology was in Mike Sanguinetti's cellular electrophysiology research lab. Mike thinks *very well*. He is the reason any of us know about I_{Kr} and I_{Ks} (formerly thought to be a single ion current). He is an immensely unassuming and generous teacher. He made me realize that science can be done by mere mortals; there is no reason you can't ask and answer your own questions.

I learned clinical electrophysiology from Warren (Sonny) Jackman. Sonny is *the* pioneer of modern interventional electrophysiology. While there is never just one person responsible for anything in science, if you had to pick a single individual as the father of ablation it would rightfully be Sonny. I have often reflected on the enormous impact that Sonny has had on EP. While he is most definitely extremely smart, he is not the only smart guy in EP; intelligence was necessary but not sufficient for the kind of impact that Sonny's had. His most important trait is intellectual tenacity. More than anyone else in my life, Sonny taught me to think *well*. I realized through Sonny that analytical thinking isn't a talent, it's a skill; it requires energy and discipline and it yields tremendous rewards.

It is only in the last six years that I've come to realize that cardiac electrophysiology is just one of many complex non-linear dynamic systems. Jason Bates taught me about complex systems and how they relate to EP. Within a week of our meeting we began to create a computer model of cardiac electrical propagation. That meeting has definitely changed my intellectual horizons more than any other meeting in my life.

It is hard to adequately express the extent of my appreciation for the advice and influence of my mentor Burt Sobel. Burt, who sadly passed away recently, was an inspiration and a master advisor. My thinking was disorganized before I met Burt. He taught me to focus. Burt combined a sharp mind with a burning curiosity, and a perpetually youthful enthusiasm with an appreciation for the elegance of ideas.

The content of this book owes a great deal to Sonny Jackman, its existence to Burt Sobel.

I'd like to thank Wendy Miner for her many, many hours of help in preparing the manuscript. I also thank my wife, Amy Spector, for the many, many hours she let me put into this book.

Peter Spector

About the companion website

This book is accompanied by a companion website:

www.wiley.com/go/spector/cardiac_electrophysiology

The website includes:

- 23 videos that demonstrate the concepts explained in the chapters
- The videos are cited throughout the text. Look out for the 👁

Many of the stills and videos throughout this text are from VisibleEP (an interactive virtual EP lab). To find out more about purchasing VisibleEP software please visit the website (http://www.VisibleEP.com). All purchasers of the VisibleEP software receive a bonus interactive edition of this book with learning materials including quizzes and exercises designed to allow students to test and re-inforce their understanding of the principles and concepts presented throughout the book.

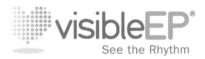

PART I

Third-person omniscient (how we would see EP if we could *see* EP)

We are taught about the heart in the same way that we are taught many topics in science. Texts tell us a fully evolved story; we are left with the impression that this story represents objective fact. The reality is that our field's current understanding of cardiac electrophysiology (EP) is cobbled together from a long series of observations, hypotheses, experiments, and their interpretations. Our present conception of how electrophysiology "works" is just the most recent state of an ever-evolving set of theories. We could retell the story as it actually evolved; recounting each conception and the subsequent observations that led us to re-categorize them as "mis"-conceptions … repeat. Telling the story this way is a great approach to teaching *research*. It is a relatively inefficient way to introduce new students to EP. Instead, like most texts, the first part of this book is told as if we *know* exactly how things work (from ion channels to arrhythmia mechanisms). I often describe

this perspective as "God's-eye view," because it presupposes (or pretends) that we have direct knowledge of the heart. My son, in high school at the time, explained to me that this narrative voice has a name: the third-person omniscient. **Part I** of *Understanding Clinical Cardiac Electrophysiology* provides a framework within which we can organize this information as we digest it.

In reality, as clinicians, we will never *see* the heart's electrical activity. Nor do we directly see the heart's anatomy. Instead we gather indirect data (e.g., x-ray, electrograms, and ultrasound) and we *deduce* what must "really" be happening in the heart. **Part II** of this book is told from the clinician's-eye view. The clinician's view is how we will actually experience EP. We gather data; we combine the data with our understanding of electrophysiology principles (Part I) and with the rules of logic; and from these we formulate a working hypothesis about what our patient's heart is doing.

Understanding Clinical Cardiac Electrophysiology: A Conceptually Guided Approach, First Edition. Peter Spector.
© 2016 John Wiley & Sons, Inc. Published 2016 by John Wiley & Sons, Inc.
Companion website: www.wiley.com/go/spector/cardiac_electrophysiology

Ion channels

Clinical electrophysiologists concern themselves with the normal and pathologic spread of activation through the walls of the heart. It is not immediately apparent that the person who finds this a fascinating intellectual pursuit will or should concern themselves with the details of ion channels, action potentials, and cellular electrophysiology. In fact, the clinical electrophysiologist need not memorize the *details* of cellular EP, but must understand the *functional consequences* that cellular EP has on tissue EP. As with all matters scientific, electrophysiology is a multi-scale phenomenon. This means that the behavior of the heart at the highest level (the whole heart) results from the individual and ensemble behavior of the components of which the heart is made (cells, ion channels, etc.). One need not understand the details of *how* the lower scales produce their behavior but must understand *what* those behaviors are. (There are many ways to skin a cat; regardless of the details, the cat no longer has skin.)

The approach taken in this chapter is to present those parts of cellular electrophysiology which are relevant to tissue physiology.[1]

At the tissue level we are concerned with **impulse formation** and **impulse conduction**. These two phenomena underlie normal and abnormal automaticity, normal and diseased conduction (within and between chambers), as well as reentrant arrhythmias (including fibrillation). Let's look then at the cellular physiology that underlies these phenomena.

---

[1] You can skip this chapter … but I'll think less of you.

How does a cell become electrically active?

Prior to the expenditure of energy there is no voltage or ion concentration gradient across the cell membrane. The inside and outside of the cell are separated by a lipid bilayer (the membrane) (Figure 1.1). The importance of the lipid is that it makes the membrane hydrophobic; therefore water and ions cannot cross the membrane. Various proteins are embedded in the membrane, spanning from the cell's interior to its exterior. One of these proteins is $Na^+K^+ATPase$, a pump that uses energy derived from adenosine triphosphate (ATP) to push Na^+ ions out of the cell and K^+ ions into the cell. By virtue of this energy expenditure a gradient is established in which Na^+ concentration is much higher outside the cell and K^+ concentration is much higher inside the cell (Figure 1.2). It is the nature of the universe that things tend toward maximum entropy (or disorganization). The result is that if order/organization is established (which requires energy), absent the continued expenditure of energy that order will tend to return to a state of disorder/disorganization. In our story this means that ions do not "want" to be segregated; all else being equal they will tend to travel down their concentration gradient, re-establishing equilibrium. The hydrophobic lipid bilayer membrane, however, prevents ions from crossing and reaching equilibrium. Here is where **ion channels** enter the story. Ion channels are proteins that span the membrane; they do so because they have a hydrophobic region which faces the membrane and a hydrophilic center (hole) which can allow passage

---

Understanding Clinical Cardiac Electrophysiology: A Conceptually Guided Approach, First Edition. Peter Spector.
© 2016 John Wiley & Sons, Inc. Published 2016 by John Wiley & Sons, Inc.
Companion website: www.wiley.com/go/spector/cardiac_electrophysiology

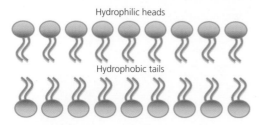

Figure 1.1 Lipid bilayer. Charged ions cannot cross the cell membrane; they are repelled by the hydrophobic lipid "tails."

of ions.[2] Ion channels, by virtue of their particular physical structure, allow passage of specific ions; not just any ion type can pass through any ion channel (e.g., Na^+ ions can pass through Na^+ channels but not K^+ channels).[3] The details of *how* this ion selectivity is achieved is critical for understanding ion channels, but irrelevant for studying tissue physiology; *that* ion channels have selectivity is critical to understanding tissue physiology. If these hydrophilic "holes" in the membrane were always open,[4] ions would always travel down their concentration gradient until equilibrium was restored. Ion channels can be either open or closed (as a result of physical changes in their shape). Whenever they are open current will flow, until or unless there are no forces to move the ions.

Let's follow imaginary K^+ ions after the Na^+K^+ATPase has created a concentration gradient and immediately after the K^+ channels have changed to the open state. The K^+ ions adjacent to the pore "feel the pull" of their concentration gradient driving them out of the cell (Figure 1.3). The pore, which lets them pass, does not allow an associated anion to cross with them. The result is that with each K^+ ion that traverses the membrane there is an increasing imbalance of charge across the membrane (one more positive charge outside than inside). This charge separation results in a voltage gradient. Having crossed the membrane, the forces acting on K^+ ions have changed; there is still an outward force generated by the concentration gradient, *and* now there is an

---

[2] It turns out that the pore of ion channels is more complex than a watery hole allowing ions to pass (if it was there would be little ion selectivity beyond "anything smaller than …"). True to my word from the introduction to this chapter, we will ignore the details as they are not relevant to the *behavior* of the pore.

[3] Although no ion channels have absolute selectivity.

[4] And if there were no other forces affecting ion flow (e.g., potential gradient).

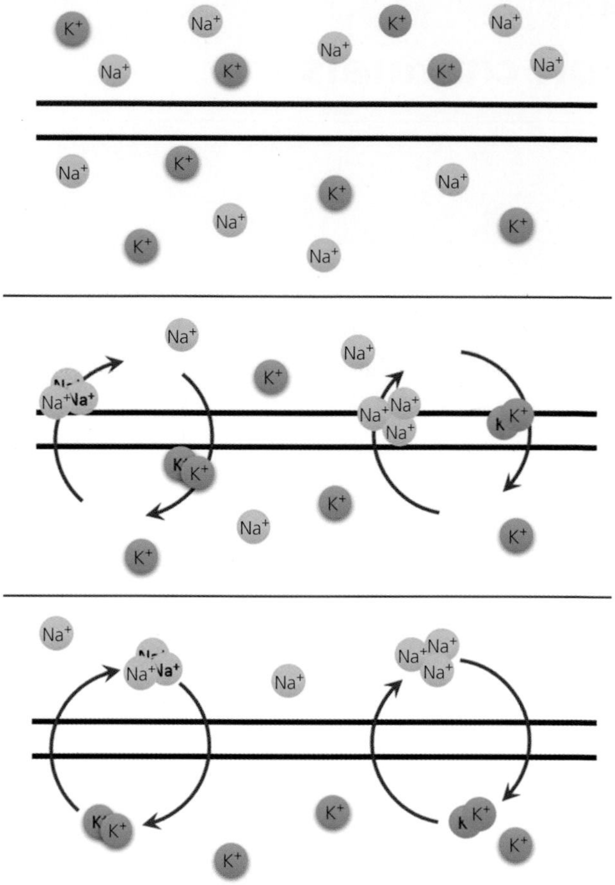

Figure 1.2 Creation of an ion concentration gradient. (Top) Without the sodium potassium pump (Na^+K^+ATPase) there is equal distribution of ions on both sides of the membrane (represented by the horizontal lines). (Middle and bottom) Na^+K^+ATPase moves Na^+ ions out of, and K^+ ions into, the cell, establishing concentration gradients for both of these ions.

inward force generated by the voltage gradient.[5] At this point the concentration-gradient force is greater than the opposing voltage force, so K^+ ions continue to flow out of the cell (albeit a little less avidly). As this flow continues the voltage gradient (and hence voltage force) grows. The concentration gradient for all intents and purposes remains unchanged (because the volumes in and out of the cell are so large compared with the actual number of ions that move). So the outward force remains fixed while the opposing inward force grows. Flow will slow until eventually the forces are balanced (equal and opposite) and there is no more *net* K^+ flow. A steady state is reached; any movement of more K^+ out of the cell will cause the

---

[5] The inside of the cell is now at a negative voltage relative to the outside, and K^+ ions are positively charged.

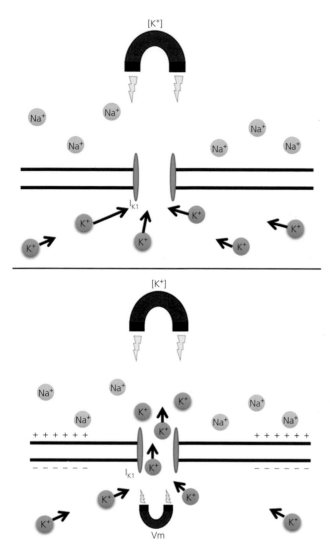

Figure 1.3 Electrochemical gradient. (Top) Once I$_{K1}$ channels open, allowing K$^+$ to move across the membrane, the K$^+$ concentration gradient pulls K$^+$ *out of* the cell. (Bottom) As K$^+$ leaves the cell (without any anions) a voltage gradient begins to develop; this exerts an *inward* force on K$^+$, reducing the net outward force. K$^+$ will continue to flow down its concentration gradient until the voltage gradient exactly offsets the concentration gradient; this voltage is called the equilibrium potential (there is no longer any *net* flow of K$^+$).

(2) the channel resistance. This is equivalent to Ohm's law, *V* = *IR*; in our case *V*, the driving force, isn't just voltage, it is the electro*chemical* gradient; *I* is ion flow and *R* is channel resistance.[6]

So far we have a pretty boring cell. What makes cellular electrophysiology so interesting is that there are multiple different types of ion channels whose dynamic gating behaviors are interdependent. It's time to discuss what controls the ion channels' open/closed state. Channels have what is described as a "gate," which can be open, allowing flow, or closed, precluding it (channel opening is called *activation* and closing is called *deactivation*). In some channel types the signal that controls the gate's position is the membrane voltage (voltage-gated channels);[7] in other channel types it is the binding of ligands (e.g., acetylcholine) that controls gating state (ligand-gated channels). There is an additional gate that can *inactivate* the channel, such that even if the activation gate is in the open state the cell is nonetheless incapable of current flow. When this gate is closed, the cell is *inactivated*; when open, the cell has *recovered from inactivation*. The state of the inactivation gate is voltage-dependent and can, in some channels, be modulated by various factors (e.g., K$^+$ concentration). Thus cells have two "doors" in series; if either is closed, current cannot flow (Figure 1.4).

Consider for a moment a membrane with both K$^+$ and Na$^+$ channels. The gating of each channel is dependent on membrane voltage (V$_m$); Na$^+$ channels *open* when membrane voltage is greater than a particular value called the Na$^+$ **threshold potential**, and K$^+$ channels behave in the opposite way; they are *open* below a certain voltage and *closed* above it. Now let's follow our ions. We'll begin with the membrane voltage at 0; ion gradients have been established but all channels are closed.[8] Let's assume that the K$^+$ channels (and only the K$^+$ channels) open. Potassium leaves the cell, resulting in membrane depolarization. This continues until the electrochemical gradient is zero (i.e., voltage gradient

voltage gradient to become larger than the concentration gradient, the net force will become inward, and K$^+$ will move back into the cell, re-establishing equilibrium. This state of affairs is described as "clamping" the membrane at the equilibrium voltage; any current flow into or out of the cell will result in an opposing flow of K$^+$.

There are two factors that control current flow through ion channels: (1) the forces acting on the ions (the net of the concentration and voltage gradients) and

---

[6] The resistance of a single ion channel influences the single-channel ion current; the single-channel resistance and the total number of channels in a cell determine the total membrane current.

[7] The voltage sensor is a group of charged amino acids in one of the membrane-spanning portions of the channel protein. Because they are charged, these amino acids "feel" the pull of the transmembrane voltage and physically move. Because these amino acids are physically connected with the rest of the channel protein, their movement causes a conformational change, opening the pore, which then allows ions to pass.

[8] This is a fictitious state we are using for the purposes of explanation.

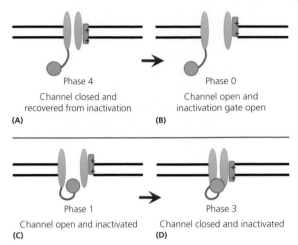

(A) Phase 4
Channel closed and
recovered from inactivation

(B) Phase 0
Channel open and
inactivation gate open

(C) Phase 1
Channel open and inactivated

(D) Phase 3
Channel closed and inactivated

Figure 1.4 Sodium channel gating. (Top left) In the resting state sodium channels are closed and their inactivation gate is open ("recovered from inactivation"). (Top right) If the membrane is depolarized to threshold the voltage sensor moves, causing a conformational change in the channel which opens the pore (activation). Because activation gating is faster than inactivation, at this point the inactivation gate remains open and sodium can enter the cell. (Bottom left) After a few milliseconds the inactivation gate closes. (Bottom right) As the membrane repolarizes the activation gate closes. With further repolarization the inactivation gate "recovers from inactivation" (opens) and the cell is prepared for the next action potential (top left).

exactly offsets concentration gradient). Under normal physiologic conditions the K^+ concentration ($[K^+]$) is ~4 meq outside and ~140 meq inside the cell. This chemical-gradient force is equal (and opposite) to a voltage gradient of ~ –85 mV (inside relative to outside). Therefore K^+ current will flow until the voltage reaches –85 mV, at which point there is no net force: steady state has been reached. If we now (magically) cause the membrane to depolarize to the Na^+ threshold potential, Na^+ channels open. Sodium ions "feel" a very strong pull into the cell (for Na^+, both the concentration gradient *and* the voltage gradient are directed inwardly). As Na^+ moves into the cell, the membrane voltage becomes less negative (the membrane *depolarizes*). The voltage gradient force on Na^+ progressively diminishes (as the inside of the membrane becomes positive relative to the outside). Sodium will continue to flow until the membrane voltage force is equal to and opposite from the concentration-gradient force (i.e., the electrochemical gradient is zero) or the resistance to Na^+ becomes infinite.[9] If the K^+ channels remained open while the Na^+

---

[9] i.e., the channels (completely) inactivate.

channels were open there would be simultaneous inward Na^+ current and outward K^+ current, the membrane voltage would depend upon the *net* flow. This, however, is not what happens. As Na^+ enters the cell, membrane potential depolarizes and K^+ channel gates close (thus whether or not there is a driving force for K^+ there is no K^+ current because K^+-resistance is infinite). It turns out the membrane never reaches Na^+ equilibrium potential because a second Na^+ channel gate (the inactivation gate) closes before equilibrium is reached.

What is the trigger that controls the inactivation gate? Interestingly the trigger for Na^+ channel opening and for Na^+ channel inactivation *is the same event*: depolarization. This seems to imply that there is *never* any Na^+ current; if the activation gate opens but the inactivation gate simultaneously closes there can never be any flow (albeit secondary to different impediments at different voltages). However, the *rate* at which the activation gate opens is much faster than the rate at which the inactivation gate closes. Therefore Na^+ current can flow after the activation gate opens and until the inactivation gate closes. If no other channel opened the membrane voltage would remain at whatever potential it reached when all the ion channels closed (it would have no way of changing). In reality there is an elegant dance in which Na^+ channels close, Ca^{++} channels slowly open (then inactivate), and a new population of K^+ channels (not those open when we started our story) begin to open. The ensemble behavior is rapid depolarization followed by slow repolarization and return to the initial state (i.e., an **action potential**). Importantly, all of this current flow and voltage change requires no direct energy expenditure; the energy was invested ahead of time when the concentration gradients were established (remember $Na^+K^+ATPase$). Once ions are separated across the membrane, dynamic changes in ion-channel gating produce fluctuating ion currents and membrane voltages. The flow of ions (while small relative to the volumes into which they flow) requires further pumping to re-establish the initial concentration conditions.

Summary

- Action potentials require no energy expenditure. They use electrochemical gradients created by the $Na^+K^+ATPase$ and open resting K^+ channels (I_{K1}).

- The membrane is a lipid bilayer impermeable to ions.
- Ion channels are proteins which provide a hole through the membrane.
- They can be open or closed, and inactivated or recovered from inactivation. These states are different physical configurations of the channel proteins.
- Control of gating can be via transmembrane voltage or ligand binding.
- The voltage sensor is a section of charged amino acids that span the membrane and are moved by transmembrane voltage. Movement of the sensor changes the channel configuration opening the pore.

- In the resting state I_{K1} is the only open channel (pretty much).
- K^+ travels down its concentration gradient. As it does so, a voltage gradient is created; steady state is reached when the voltage gradient is equal and opposite to the chemical gradient.
- K^+ concentration determines the resting membrane potential.
- I_{K1} acts as a voltage "clamp" resisting changes to membrane voltage.

The "whole point" (of cardiac electrical activity) is a phasic depolarization and repolarization *that links* to phasic release of calcium which interacts with the cell's contractile proteins. The action potential (AP) is the net voltage trajectory of the cell membrane; i.e., it results from the ensemble behavior of all the ion channels. The behaviors of the ion channels are interrelated via membrane voltage and ion gradients, with each *reacting to* the membrane voltage[1] and each *changing* the membrane voltage.

The membrane can be thought of like a boulder at the top of a hill; the action potential requires no acute energy expenditure. The separation of ions, which produces the electrochemical gradients, is created by pumps *before* the action potential. The currents are all passive, releasing the potential energy invested by the pumps.

The shape of a cell's action potential is determined by the number and properties of the ion channels in its membrane. There can be subtle variations in AP morphology throughout different regions in the heart (Figure 2.1) and even across the thickness of the heart's walls. The most prominent differences are between the "working-type" and the "pacemaker-type" myocytes (Figure 2.2). Atrial, ventricular, and His–Purkinje cells are "working-type" cells which, due to the presence of Na^+ channels, have a very rapid upstroke and very brief relative[2] refractory period. The sinus and AV nodal cells are "pacemaker-type" cells. They have a more depolarized resting membrane potential, spontaneous depolarization leading to self-excitation (hence the name), and a relatively slow upstroke (due to the presence of Ca^{++} current and the absence of Na^+ current) and a prolonged relative refractory period.

Action potential phases

Phase 4 (diastole)

The initial (and final) phase of the action potential is phase 4. Working-type cells have a large number of I_{K1} channels, which are the predominant ion channels open in the resting state. Because (essentially) the only ion channels open are K^+ channels, the resting potential is close to the equilibrium potential for K^+ *and* these cells resist depolarization (remember I_{K1}'s voltage clamping effect – Chapter 1). The presence of minimal, intrinsic, spontaneous depolarizing currents in combination with the significant voltage clamping effect of I_{K1} means that, unperturbed, these cells will remain at resting potential. They are *followers*, not leaders;[3] they depolarize only in response to external current (via gap junctions from their neighbors or as a result of electrode pacing). In pacemaker-type cells, phase 4 is not steady state; there is spontaneous depolarization which does not require external currents. This is true, in part, because their relatively small amount of I_{K1} allows them to be more easily depolarized. We will discuss pacemaker activity in Chapter 4).

Phase 0 (upstroke)

Once the membrane has reached the Na^+ channel's activation threshold, Na^+ channels open (Figure 2.3). This leads to inward Na^+ current and further membrane

---

[1] and ion concentration gradients.
[2] See below.

[3] It turns out that most cells have *some* spontaneous depolarizing currents and can therefore act as auxiliary pacemaker cells under certain circumstances.

Understanding Clinical Cardiac Electrophysiology: A Conceptually Guided Approach, First Edition. Peter Spector.
© 2016 John Wiley & Sons, Inc. Published 2016 by John Wiley & Sons, Inc.
Companion website: www.wiley.com/go/spector/cardiac_electrophysiology

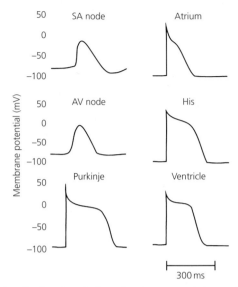

Figure 2.1 **Regional variation of action potential morphology.** AP morphology varies in the heart. It is determined by the ion channels and pumps expressed in a cell's membrane (as well as dynamic conditions like heart rate and autonomic tone).

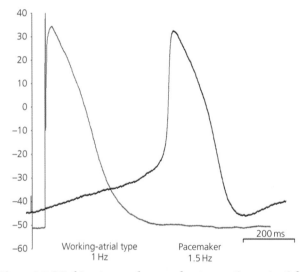

Figure 2.2 **Working-type and pacemaker-type action potentials.** Pacemaker cells are capable of spontaneous phase 4 depolarization leading to automaticity. In order for a cell to manifest spontaneous depolarization it must (1) have inward currents that are active below the threshold of Na^+ or Ca^{++} channels and (2) have *reduced* I_{K1} (outward potassium current resists depolarization).

depolarization. The I_{K1} channels that had been open at rest are inactivated and stop passing current. Inward current magnitude is large and depolarization occurs very quickly (i.e., there is a high dV/dt[4]). Meanwhile the Na^+ channel's inactivation gate closes (relatively slowly

---

[4] dV/dt is a notation from calculus that represents the English phrase "rate of change of voltage over time."

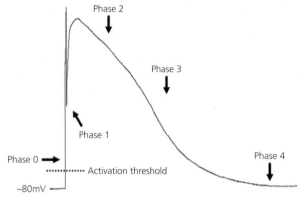

Figure 2.3 **Action potential phases.** Phase 0: Na^+ channels open once the membrane reaches Na^+ activation threshold – producing rapid depolarization. Phase 1: I_{to} opens and I_{Na} closes, causing rapid (brief) repolarization. Phase 2: I_{to} closes and I_{Ca} opens; there is a slow shift from predominantly inward currents to predominantly outward currents. Phase 3: I_{Ca} closes and I_{Kr} and I_{Ks} open, causing repolarization. Phase 4: I_{Kr} and I_{Ks} close, I_{Na} closes and recovers from inactivation, and I_{K1} opens.

compared with the rate at which the channel activated). Due to Na^+ channel inactivation the membrane never actually reaches the Na^+ reversal potential.

Phase 1 (transient repolarization)

At this point the membrane reaches the activation threshold for I_{to} (the transient outward potassium channel). Once the membrane has become permeable to potassium, K^+ travels down its electrochemical gradient out of the cell.[5] As the name implies, I_{to} is transient. Like the Na^+ channel, I_{to} activates more quickly than it inactivates, so passes current in the period of time between activation and inactivation.

Phase 2 (the "plateau")

Early in phase 0 the membrane reaches the activation threshold for the Ca^{++} channel.[6] Ca^{++} channel activation is slow (compared with Na^+ channels) but at this point inward Ca^{++} current is flowing. The combination of turning "off" I_{to} and "on" I_{Ca} causes the membrane to rebound to a more positive V_m (Figure 2.3), and thus the transition from phase 1 to phase 2 looks like a "spike-and-dome." Throughout phase 2 Ca^{++} channels are progressively inactivating and two new K^+ channels are beginning to open (I_{Kr} and I_{Ks}). The net result is a steady shift from inward to outward current and concomitant repolarization.

---

[5] With a positive V_m both voltage and K^+ gradient drive K^+ out of the cell.
[6] There are several different Ca^{++} channels; here we are talking about the "L-type" Ca^{++} channel.

Phase 3 (repolarization)

As the membrane voltage becomes more polarized, I_{Kr} and I_{Ks} begin to close and I_{K1} begins to re-open. In addition repolarization triggers recovery from inactivation of Na$^+$ (and Ca^{++}) channels. This ultimately brings us to where we started, phase 4, and the process can repeat.

The connection between ion channel physiology and tissue behavior

Having discussed the broad strokes of the action potential, let's move on to the "who cares?" part of action potentials (from the clinician's perspective). A big part of this story is the behavior of the cell's Na$^+$ channels. First, Na$^+$ current in large part determines the rate of depolarization (dV/dt). As we'll see next, we care about dV/dt because this has a large influence on the **conduction velocity** of propagation (a macroscopic behavior that clinicians most certainly care about). In addition, Na$^+$ channels are important because while they are inactivated the cell is **refractory** (i.e., cannot be re-excited regardless of membrane depolarization).

Sodium channels and conduction velocity

This is pretty straightforward. The faster a cell depolarizes the sooner there is a voltage gradient between it and its neighbors. The cell–cell voltage gradient is the driving force for spread of current between cells;[7] it is this current that brings the *next* cell to threshold. Thus the larger the I_{Na}, the faster a cell depolarizes and the faster its neighbors become activated.

Sodium channels and refractory period

At the conclusion of phase 0 the Na$^+$ channel inactivation gate closes; the cell cannot have another action potential until the inactivation gates re-open.[8] In phase 4 (resting) the Na$^+$ channel is closed and the inactivation gate is open (Figure 1.4); the cell is poised for an action potential. During phase 0 the Na$^+$ channels open and shortly thereafter their inactivation gate closes. During phase 2 Na$^+$ channels close/deactivate (their inactivation gates remain closed) (Figure 1.4).[9] At some point during phase 3, as the membrane repolarizes, Na$^+$ channel inactivation gates *begin* to open. Importantly, there is not an abrupt change from "all channels inactivated" to "all channels recovered from inactivation." The macroscopic implication is that once *some* Na$^+$ channels are recovered the cell can have an action potential; but until *all* channels have recovered the magnitude of the I_{Na} during an action potential will be reduced compared with baseline. Therefore, during this recovery period, any induced action potential will have less I_{Na} and hence will have a reduced dV/dt. The result is that action potentials elicited during the relative refractory period propagate with slower conduction velocity. There are three stages of refractoriness during an action potential: the **absolute refractory period** (when Na$^+$ channels are inactivated), the **relative refractory period** (when some Na$^+$ channels have recovered), and the **fully excitable period** (when all Na$^+$ channels have recovered from inactivation) (Figure 2.4). Because refractoriness is related to Na$^+$ channel inactivation, and because inactivation is related to membrane potential, **refractoriness is dependent**

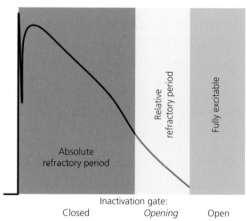

Figure 2.4 Sodium channel gating and refractoriness. Following depolarization, Na$^+$ channel inactivation gates close and the cell cannot be re-excited until the inactivation gate re-opens (absolute refractory period). As some, but not all gates recover from inactivation the cell can be re-excited, but only those channels that have recovered are available to pass current. Hence the dV/dt and conduction velocity are reduced (relative refractory period). Finally, once all channels have recovered from inactivation the cell is once again fully excitable.

[7] via gap junctions. Unlike the ion channels we've been discussing, gap junctions are essentially ungated (they're always open). One exception to this is the presence of intracellular acidosis. The result is that infarcted/ischemic cells become electrically disconnected from their neighbors.
[8] and/or the Ca^{++} channel recovers.

[9] Since the channels are already inactivated (and therefore not passing current) there is no electrical indicator that the channels have switched from open to closed.

upon action potential duration (i.e., the amount of time the membrane takes to repolarize sufficiently to recover inactivation gates).

Potassium channels and action potential duration

Now that we've identified the important role that action potential duration (APD) plays in refractoriness, let's discuss what determines APD. The cell depolarizes in response to inward currents (Na$^+$ and Ca^{++}) and it repolarizes in response to outward currents (K$^+$).[10]

Repolarization begins as Ca^{++} currents start inactivating and the "delayed rectifier" K$^+$ currents activate. The greater the magnitude of I_K the faster repolarization occurs (i.e., shorter APD) (Figure 2.5). There are several different K$^+$ channels, but the two that contribute most to understanding events at the clinical level are I_{Kr} and I_{Ks}. These were named for their respective gating kinetics: I_{Kr} has rapid gating while I_{Ks} has very slow gating (Figure 2.6). I can almost hear your eyelids drooping at the mention of "kinetics" but you care and I'll tell you why. Because I_{Kr} activates and deactivates rapidly, its amplitude is *not rate-dependent* (Figure 2.7). I_{Ks} is different: (1) it has slower kinetics and (2) *not all I_{Ks} channels open* during an AP. The population of I_{Ks} channels possesses what is referred to as *repolarization reserve*: only a portion of all I_{Ks} channels open during an AP, so there are more that *could* open. Finally, because

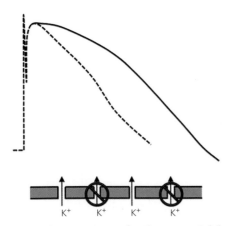

Figure 2.5 Potassium current and action potential duration. The membrane repolarizes as outward K$^+$ currents exceed inward currents. When fewer K$^+$ channels are available (e.g., in the presence of an antiarrhythmic medication) it takes longer for the membrane to repolarize (i.e., the APD is increased).

[10] combined with decreasing inward currents.

deactivation is slow, if there is insufficient time between APs not all I_{Ks} channels have a chance to close before the next AP opens more I_{Ks} channels. The combined effect is "stacking" of I_{Ks} at rapid rates; $\mathbf{I_{Ks}}$ **amplitude is *rate-dependent*** (Figure 2.8).

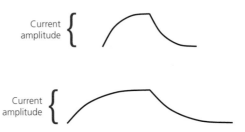

Figure 2.6 $\mathbf{I_{Kr}}$ and $\mathbf{I_{Ks}}$ kinetics. (Top) I_{Kr} rapidly opens and deactivates/inactivates. (Bottom) I_{Ks} slowly opens and deactivates/inactivates.

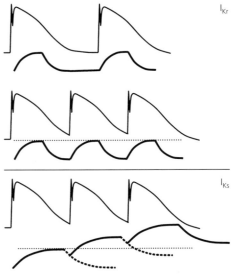

Figure 2.7 Effects of rate on $\mathbf{I_{Kr}}$ and $\mathbf{I_{Ks}}$ amplitude. (Top) I_{Kr} can fully recover even at rapid rates; (Bottom) at rapid rates I_{Ks} (1) is incompletely activated and (2) cannot fully deactivate between beats. As a result I_{Ks} current amplitude progressively increases at fast rates (I_{Ks} "stacking").

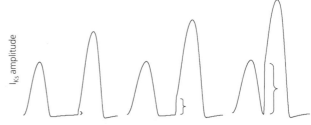

Figure 2.8 $\mathbf{I_{Ks}}$ stacking. Here we see that as diastolic interval decreases (faster rates) K$^+$ current amplitude does not reach zero between beats so net current increases with rate.

Who cares? There are two implications of this rate-dependence. First, at faster heart rates the diastolic interval is decreased;[11] and (because I_{Ks} is rate-dependent) this produces more repolarizing current and a shorter APD. This rate-dependence is called **restitution** (Figure 2.9). Restitution allows the heart to be excited more frequently ... when it's excited more frequently. Second (and very importantly), it means that at rapid rates I_{Kr} contributes less to repolarization than it does at slower rates (Figure 2.10).

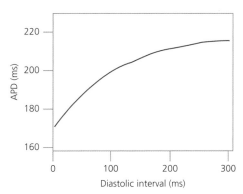

Figure 2.9 Action potential duration restitution. As heart rate increases (diastolic interval decreases) APD decreases (in part due to stacking of I_{Ks}).

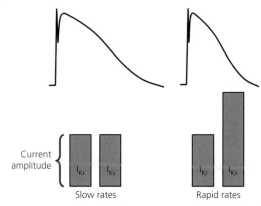

Figure 2.10 I_{Kr}/I_{Ks} ratio as a function of rate. Due to stacking, I_{Ks} accounts for a greater proportion of repolarizing current at rapid rates. This has important implications for antiarrhythmic medications.

Based upon the physiology described above:

Question: If you could design an "ideal" antiarrhythmic drug (maximally antiarrhythmic and minimally pro-arrhythmic) would it be better to block I_{Kr} or I_{Ks}? Why?

Answer: Imagine a drug that blocks I_{Ks}. Such a drug will have its greatest impact on APD/refractoriness at rapid rates (because I_{Ks} has a proportionally greater influence on APD at rapid rates). This is just what you'd want in an antiarrhythmic drug – alter electrophysiology at fast rates (to prevent tachycardia) but not at slow rates (to reduce pro-arrhythmia).[12] If, on the other hand, you give a drug that blocks I_{Kr}, that drug will have its greatest effect on APD at slow rates (because the *impact* of I_{Kr} on repolarization is greatest at slow rates). Thus I_{Kr} blockers have a greater effect at slow rates (increasing their potential for pro-arrhythmia) and are less effective at fast rates (decreasing their antiarrhythmic efficacy) (Figure 2.11). I_{Kr} blockers are described as having "reverse"[13] use-dependence; i.e., they are less effective at slower rates.

Question: What time is the most sensitive for identifying the QT-prolonging effect of I_{Kr}-blocking drugs (e.g., dofetilide or sotalol)?

Answer: When we observe patients on telemetry during loading of a QT-prolonging drug we are looking for any indication of a dangerous impact on *ventricular* electrophysiology; we are not watching for evidence of efficacy with regard to atrial electrophysiology. Thus the "best" time to look for QT prolongation refers to the most sensitive time. Due to restitution, the greatest impact of an I_{Kr}-blocking drug is following the longest diastolic interval. Long diastolic intervals are often seen due to variable conduction of AF (Figure 2.12) and upon spontaneous conversion of AF. In addition we can look at the "magnitude" of pro-arrhythmic indicators. QT prolongation alone is less concerning than QT prolongation with an associated premature ventricular contraction (PVC) arising from the T wave ... which is less concerning than prolonged QT and a PVC on the T that initiates non-sustained VT or torsade.

---

[11] One can divide the excitation cycle into a systolic and diastolic component. The systolic component is the action potential; the diastolic component is the period between repolarization and the next depolarization. As the heart beats more quickly the diastolic interval is reduced *more than* the APD is reduced. The consequence is a shorter amount of time for recovery from inactivation.

[12] As we will see, APD prolongation can lead to triggered firing and torsade de pointes.

[13] The word "reverse" is in quotes because I_{Kr} blockers bind with the channel *more* at fast rates (i.e., they are actually *use*-dependent). However, because the impact of I_{Kr} blockade is diminished at fast rates (due to the increased magnitude of I_{Ks}) the *effectiveness* of I_{Kr} blockers is reverse use-dependent.

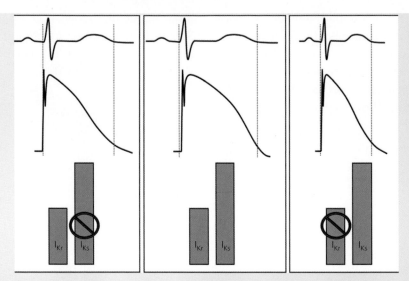

Figure 2.11 Differential effects of I$_{Kr}$ and I$_{Ks}$ blockade. (Middle) As heart rate increases the role of I$_{Ks}$ in repolarizing the membrane increases (relative to I$_{Kr}$). (Left) If we block I$_{Ks}$ we are blocking a larger proportion of repolarizing current and will have a large effect on APD (and hence QT). (Right) If we block I$_{Kr}$ we are blocking a smaller proportion of the repolarizing current and hence have a lesser effect on APD (and QT) than block of I$_{Ks}$ would have.

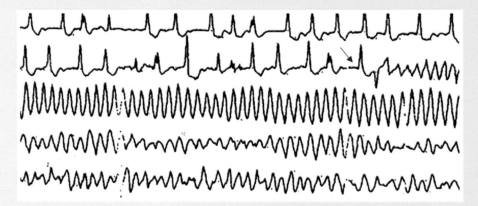

Figure 2.12 Long-short interval precipitates torsade de pointes. An early beat followed by a compensatory pause (arrow) produces increased QT prolongation; a triggered beat (R-on-T) results in initiation of torsade de pointes.

Clinical correlation

Wide complex tachycardia in the emergency room

A 57-year-old man presents to the emergency room (ER) for evaluation of shortness of breath. He has a history of asthma and prostate cancer. He was transported to the ER by paramedics who report that he was initially awake and anxious with a blood pressure of 180/100 mmHg, a heart rate of 120 bpm, and a respiratory rate of 32. They started an IV and 100% oxygen by nasal cannula, and obtained a rhythm strip which revealed sinus tachycardia at a rate of 120 bpm. Upon presentation

to the ER he was sitting upright, was diaphoretic, and was in respiratory distress. He otherwise had an unremarkable exam. His EKG is shown in Figure 2.13.

What is your interpretation of the rhythm? What would you do next?

In this patient's case, he was given a bolus of 100 mg of lidocaine (this was in the 1990s). He immediately became asystolic. Why? What would you do next?

He was given calcium, remained refractory to all therapy, and was declared dead one hour after arrival in the ER.

A postmortem examination revealed a non-ruptured dissecting thoracic aortic aneurysm and acute tubular

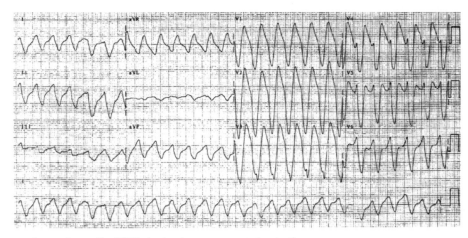

Figure 2.13 Wide complex tachycardia. EKG obtained upon presentation to the emergency room.

necrosis. The initial blood sample from the ER returned revealing a potassium level of 9.4 and a creatinine of 18.2.

Lidocaine and hyperkalemia

In order to understand what happened in this case (and to see an example of how knowledge of cellular electrophysiology can help us in the clinical arena) we must first discuss how lidocaine works.

Lidocaine blocks sodium channels in the inactivated state; i.e., it binds to the channel protein when it is in the inactivated conformation more readily than when it is in the recovered conformation. If you think about this it seems, at first, puzzling how this could have any antiarrhythmic effect. "If the channel is inactivated, it's already *not* passing any current … so how can blocking it change electrophysiology?" The answer lies in the effect that lidocaine binding has on the **next** beat (i.e., the one after lidocaine has become bound). Because lidocaine preferentially binds to the channel in the inactivated state, as the channel recovers from inactivation it is no longer as receptive to lidocaine binding, which therefore dissociates from the channel. This dissociation *takes time*. Until lidocaine unbinds, the channel cannot pass Na^+ current. Therefore the refractory period includes the time that the channel is inactivated *plus* the time required for lidocaine to dissociate; lidocaine confers **post-repolarization refractoriness**.

Now let's consider the effect that systemic hyperkalemia has on lidocaine binding. As discussed in Chapter 1, hyperkalemia results in membrane

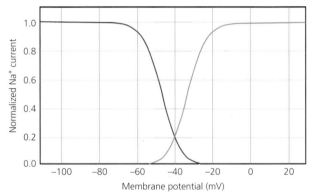

Figure 2.14 Voltage-dependence of sodium channel gating. Sodium channel activation (green) and steady-state inactivation (red) curves.

depolarization (the potassium concentration gradient is reduced, and therefore the voltage gradient that offsets it is reduced – this voltage is the resting membrane potential). Membrane depolarization increases the percentge of sodium channels that are in the inactivated state (inactivation is voltage-dependent: Figure 2.14). As mentioned above, lidocaine preferentially binds to Na^+ channels in the inactivated state, hence **lidocaine binding is increased by hyperkalemia**. Because the resting membrane potential is higher (more depolarized), lidocaine remains bound to a greater portion of Na^+ channels. Thus, when activation does occur there are fewer Na^+ channels available to pass current, so membrane depolarization occurs more slowly (decreased dV/dt). This in turn decreases conduction velocity.

Lidocaine and ischemia

In the days before widespread use of amiodarone, lidocaine was very commonly used to treat ischemic ventricular tachycardia. The logic of lidocaine for treatment of ischemic arrhythmias is related to the interactions between hyperkalemia and lidocaine binding. When a cell is inadequately perfused for a sufficient period, that cell dies and its membrane integrity fails. The "stuff" that was inside the cell now leaks into the extracellular space. Amongst that stuff are enzymes like creatine phosphokinase (CPK) and troponin (which is why these rise in the setting of infarction). The concentration of K^+ inside the cell (~140 meq) is much higher than outside the cell thanks to the $Na^+K^+ATPase$ (see Chapter 1). A large quantity of K^+ leaks into the interstitial space around infarcted cells. The $[K^+]$ remains elevated in the vicinity of the infarct, for the same reason that the cells died in the first place, namely inadequate blood flow, which diminishes the ability to "wash away" K^+. Thus local $[K^+]$ is extremely high (~15 meq), decreasing as one moves farther from the infarct zone. This creates the substrate for ventricular arrhythmias in several ways. Living cells, in the zone surrounding the central infarcted cells, are exposed to the highest $[K^+]$, are markedly depolarized, and are unexcitable. This region is surrounded by a region of lower $[K^+]$ where cells are capable of excitation but with lower dV/dt and slower conduction velocity. This provides the ideal substrate for reentry (dead cells creating an obstacle around which reentry can occur and a zone of slowed conduction (increased $[K^+]$) decreasing the likelihood that the wave front will hit its refractory tail). In addition, living cells in the zone bathed in elevated $[K^+]$ are depolarized and more susceptible to abnormal automaticity (see Chapter 4). The presence of a reentrant circuit, plus early extra systoles, enhances the likelihood of reentry (trigger and circuit).

In focal hyperkalemia (ischemia), as opposed to systemic hyperkalemia, the pro-arrhythmic effect of hyperkalemia is spatially localized (to the peri-infarct zone). Lidocaine becomes a "silver bullet" having a preferential pharmacologic effect in the pathologic zone (greater $[K^+]$, membrane depolarization, enhanced Na^+ channel inactivation). This is the ideal antiarrhythmic setting: pharmacologic influence targeted to abnormal cells while relatively sparing healthy cells. In contrast, during systemic hyperkalemia the lidocaine effect is diffuse.

Long QT syndrome

Long QT syndrome, an inherited or acquired predisposition to sudden cardiac death, is an excellent example of how understanding cellular electrophysiology can be relevant to macroscopic/clinical electrophysiology. In order to understand long QT, why it occurs and how to treat it, we must explore cellular repolarization in a little more depth.

The QT interval is not equal to, but is proportional to, the APD of ventricular myocytes. Specifically the onset of the QRS marks the time at which the first ventricular cells depolarize (while other ventricular cells remain at rest). This results in a voltage gradient across the ventricles which produces a deflection on the surface EKG. The end of the QRS is the point at which all ventricular myocytes have depolarized and there is no longer a gradient[14] (hence the ST segment is flat). The T-wave onset marks the time at which the first ventricular cells begin to *repolarize*, and the end of the T wave marks the time when all cells have repolarized.[15] On average, if the ventricular myocytes have a longer APD the delay from depolarization to repolarization will be greater and hence the QT interval will be longer. The QT is thus proportional to the APD (but is also influenced by conduction time).

The APD is determined by the balance of depolarizing and repolarizing currents. As phase 2 progresses to phase 3, inward currents diminish while outward currents increase, leading to repolarization. Anything that decreases inward currents or increases outward currents will decrease APD. In fact ion channel abnormalities that increase inward currents and those that decrease outward currents have both been identified in patients with congenital long QT.

Why does QT prolongation have the potential to be pro-arrhythmic? Interestingly the problem begins with release of Ca^{++} from the sarcoplasmic reticulum (SR). I say "interestingly" because at first glance it seems that

---

[14] Cells are not at resting potential, but they are all at the *same* potential.

[15] In fact the QRS begins shortly *after* the first myocytes depolarize. Deflection is only seen on the surface once a sufficiently large number of cells have depolarized to generate a signal large enough to be detected at the body surface.

SR Ca^{++} release would have no electrical effect. The SR membrane isn't the cell membrane (so any voltage gradient ought to be across the SR membrane). More importantly, unlike when Ca^{++} is released from ion channels, when it's released from the SR it is accompanied by anions. Thus there is no net charge movement with SR Ca^{++} release. So why is SR Ca^{++} release electrogenic? The answer relates to what happens *in response to* SR Ca^{++} release.

Calcium current, via L-type calcium channels, initiates SR Ca^{++} release. After passing through the contractile proteins this Ca^{++} is pumped back into the SR (by the SR calcium pump, **SERCA**). Once initiated, the time course of this "*calcium transient*" (transient increase in intracellular calcium concentration) *is not directly dependent on the membrane potential*. In the setting of significant APD prolongation, the APD can exceed the duration of the calcium transient (Figure 2.15).

There is a period, after Ca^{++} has been resorbed into the SR, during which intracellular Ca^{++} concentration is low while membrane potential is high (gray bar in

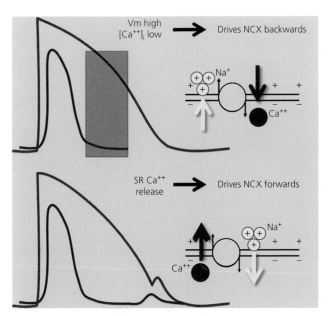

Figure 2.15 Membrane voltage, intracellular calcium transient, and triggered firing. (Top) When the APD is prolonged without an associated change in the duration of the intracellular calcium transient, the sodium–calcium exchanger (NCX) is driven "backward." (Bottom) The increased calcium causes release of calcium from the sarcoplasmic reticulum, which drives the NCX "forward." Because three sodium ions (+3) are exchanged for one calcium ion (+2) there is a net current in the direction that sodium moves. In this case the NCX creates an inward depolarizing current (an early after-depolarization).

Figure 2.15). Under these conditions the net effect of the Ca^{++}, Na$^+$, and voltage gradients drives the sodium–calcium exchanger (NCX) backward (sending Ca^{++} into and Na$^+$ out of the cell). This, in turn, causes a rise in Ca^{++} near the ryanodine receptor, which triggers a second SR Ca^{++} release. The balance of forces on the NCX now drives it forward, causing a net shift of one positive charge **into** the cell,[16] i.e., a depolarizing current (Figure 2.15). If this depolarization occurs after the cell has recovered from refractoriness, and is sufficient to bring the cell to threshold, a new action potential will be triggered (hence the name **triggered firing**).

Summary

- Action potential phases: rest (4), depolarization (0), early repolarization (1), plateau (2), repolarization (3).
- Phase 4: At rest only I_{K1} is open.
- Phase 0: When V_m reaches I_{Na} activation threshold, sodium channels open. Na$^+$ enters the cell (down its voltage and concentration gradient). V_m depolarizes rapidly. K$^+$ channels close. The threshold for I_{Na} inactivation is essentially the same as the threshold for activation. Because inactivation kinetics are much slower than activation kinetics, there is a transient inward Na$^+$ current.
- Phase 1: I_{to} transiently opens, causing rapid repolarization.
- Phase 2: I_{to} inactivates (same threshold as, slower kinetics than, activation) and I_{Ca} opens (its activation threshold is close to I_{Na} but its activation kinetics are slower than the Na$^+$ channel's).
- Phase 3: I_{Ca} begins to inactivate (more slowly than it activates). I_{Kr} and I_{Ks} open, causing repolarization.
- Phase 4: Return to rest. Repolarization closes I_{Kr} and I_{Ks}; I_{Na} recovers from inactivation; I_{Ca} recovers from inactivation (but this takes some time, causing post-repolarization refractoriness of calcium-channel-dependent cells); I_{K1} re-opens.
- Sodium channels determine dV/dt and hence conduction velocity. Recovery from inactivation of sodium channels determines refractory period. The relative

---

[16] Because the NCX swaps one calcium ion (two positive charges) for three sodium ions (three positive charges) the net result is one charge flowing in the direction that sodium flows.

(partial) refractory period occurs when some, but not all, sodium channels have recovered from inactivation.

- K$^+$ channels (largely) determine APD (which in turn determines refractory period).
- I$_{Kr}$ has rapid kinetics (no change in I$_{Kr}$ with rate).
- I$_{Ks}$ has slow kinetics and incomplete opening with a single AP. Therefore at fast heart rates I$_{Ks}$ "stacks," causing shortened APD.

- At rapid rates I$_{Ks}$ is responsible for a greater proportion of total repolarizing current, and therefore I$_{Kr}$ blockers have "reverse use-dependence." Reverse use-dependence confers a poor toxic/therapeutic ratio and thus can be pro-arrhythmic (maximum effect at slow rates and minimum effect at rapid rates).

3

Propagation

To understand the behavior of cardiac tissue we must understand how each cell behaves and how cells are connected.

The set of "rules" that govern tissue behavior are relatively simple, yet because of the number of cells and the parallel nature of their interactions, the behavior of the tissue as a whole can be quite complex. Despite the wide variety of activation patterns that the heart can manifest, understanding the rules that govern this behavior allows one to easily predict how the heart will behave under most circumstances.

Cell capacitance

Cells become excited when they are depolarized to their threshold for activation. Non-pacemaker cells remain at resting potential until exogenous current results in their depolarization. This current can enter from neighboring cells (via gap junctions) or from an external electronic pacing stimulus; in order to result in activation, this current must be sufficient to cause depolarization to the activation threshold. Once threshold is reached, the cell generates its own depolarizing current (via Na^+ or Ca^{++} channels). We refer to excited cells as the current **source**, and the neighboring unexcited cells that they provide depolarizing current to as the **sink**.

In order to understand the dynamics that govern this process we must consider all its components. First, *current* is not *voltage*. So when current enters a cell, the amount of voltage change that results depends upon the cell's *capacitance*. This can be thought of as a conversion rate, "how much depolarization is a unit of current worth?" Each cell has its own conversion rate. A cell's capacitance is related to the area of its membrane. Imagine a square patch of membrane; its voltage is a function of the number of charges on each side of the membrane. When current is delivered to the cell, charges are added to one or the other surface of the membrane. The transmembrane voltage is a function of the charge separation *per unit area* across that membrane. Therefore a cell with larger surface area will depolarize less than one with a smaller area, in response to the same current. A cell's capacitance is therefore influenced by its size.

One can think of the cell as a bucket; the radius of the bucket is analogous to its capacitance, the *height* of water in the bucket corresponds to the cell's voltage, and the water itself corresponds to current (Figure 3.1). When current flows into the bucket its voltage level rises. In response to a given amount of water flow, the water level will rise less in a wider bucket than a narrower bucket (Figure 3.2).[1]

Imagine that when the level reaches the threshold-height it begins to magically fill with its own current (after reaching threshold, current enters the cell via the transmembrane ion channels; prior to reaching threshold, current enters only via gap junctions). Now, imagine a cell that is connected to a second cell via gap junctions (Figure 3.3). This is like our first sink bucket connected by a hose *at its bottom* to a second sink bucket. As current flows into the first bucket, some of that current raises the voltage of the first bucket, but a portion of the current flows to the next bucket, raising *its* level.

Thus when two unexcited cells are connected to each other, more depolarizing current is required per unit increase of voltage (Figure 3.3). You can also see that if the resistance through the gap junctions between the two cells is very low, current will flow (between buckets)

---

[1] Think of pouring a cup of water into another cup vs. pouring it into a bath tub: the water will be deeper when poured into the cup.

Understanding Clinical Cardiac Electrophysiology: A Conceptually Guided Approach, First Edition. Peter Spector.
© 2016 John Wiley & Sons, Inc. Published 2016 by John Wiley & Sons, Inc.
Companion website: www.wiley.com/go/spector/cardiac_electrophysiology

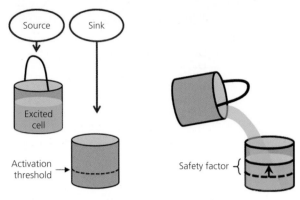

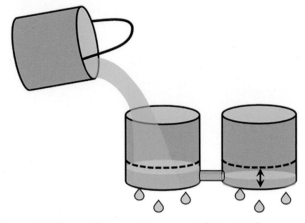

Figure 3.1 Source and sink. Source is the current available to depolarize unexcited cells. Sink is the net current required to depolarize unexcited cells to threshold.

Figure 3.4 Outward current increases sink size. In the presence of outward current (e.g., I_{K1}), source current causes less depolarization.

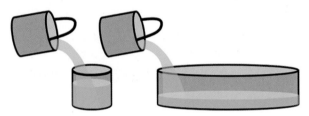

Figure 3.2 Sink size varies. If the amount of source current is unchanged while the size of the sink increases, the membrane will depolarize less.

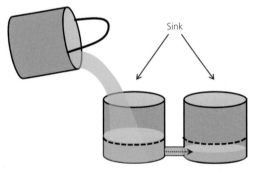

Figure 3.3 Intercellular coupling increases sink size. As cells are electrically connected, the source current is distributed to a greater number of cells.

more rapidly. If the resistance is low enough the voltage increase in both cells will be identical (i.e., half the current is going to each and the two together behave as if they were one bucket that is double in size).

Now consider what happens if the cell develops outward current in response to membrane depolarization (remember the "voltage clamping" effect of K^+ channels). This outward current will oppose the depolarizing effect of the inward current. In our bucket analogy this would be like a bucket with a hole in the bottom: as

current flows in, a portion results in the level rising (depolarization) while another portion leaks through the hole in the bottom, diminishing the amount that the level rises (Figure 3.4).

What about the rate of depolarization? For any given depolarizing current the membrane will depolarize more slowly if: (1) the cell membrane area is large, (2) the cell has many gap junctions to many neighbors, and/or (3) the cell has a lot of open K^+ channels.

To get an intuitive feel for tissue conduction, imagine a line of buckets in a row. As one bucket fills, it passes current to its neighbor, which passes current to its neighbor (etc.). The force driving current from one cell to the next is the voltage gradient (here represented by the difference in water height between the buckets). So as a cell slowly depolarizes, a small gradient develops between it and its neighbor; therefore a small amount of current flows to the neighbor. When the first cell reaches threshold its voltage rapidly increases (depolarizes) via inward Na^+ or Ca^{++} current. The voltage gradient between this, now excited, cell and its neighbor is abruptly increased, resulting in more rapid current flow to the neighbor. Thus the lateral flow of current between cells is slow (before threshold is reached) and then rapid (after threshold has been reached). Because intercellular current flow is so much more rapid between an excited cell and its neighbor, the rate of intercellular current flow is directly influenced by how quickly cells reach threshold. Intercellular resistance has a complex influence on conduction velocity. When the resistance between the source cell and sink cell is low, current will flow more quickly and hence the sink will reach threshold and become excited more quickly (increasing conduction velocity). On the other hand, if the resistance between *sink cells* is low, then source current will be spread out through a larger number of sink cells and depolarization to threshold will occur more slowly (decreasing conduction velocity). Here's the tricky part: cells are alternately sink cells (pre-excitation) and then source cells (post-excitation) with each passing wave. Thus the intercellular resistance between source and sink is the same as that between sink and sink. There is a fine balance between an intercellular resistance that is too low and one that is too high.

To recap from last chapter: if the inward current is large, depolarization occurs quickly; with smaller current, depolarization is slower. Sodium channels result in much more rapid upstroke velocity (dV/dt) than Ca^{++} channels because of their relatively larger current amplitude.[2] A cell with more Na^+ channels has larger Na^+ current and a more rapid dV/dt than a cell with fewer Na^+ channels. If some percentage of a cell's Na^+ channels are inactivated, i.e., not passing current, the net rate of depolarization is reduced. This can occur with antiarrhythmic agents that block Na^+ channels or with any factors that result in resting membrane depolarization (which increases the percentage of Na^+ channels that are in the inactivated state).

Source–sink relationship

Based upon the descriptions above you can see that if the source is large (relative to the sink) two things will happen: (1) the *likelihood* that the sink cells will reach threshold is high, and (2) the *rate* at which they reach threshold is high. Thus, the source/sink ratio determines both the **safety factor** (the amount of current beyond that which is required to reach threshold: Figure 3.1) and the conduction velocity (CV) (which is proportional to the time required to reach threshold). As the source/sink ratio decreases, both the safety factor and the CV are reduced, ultimately resulting in conduction failure (due to failure to reach threshold). Because depolarized cells comprise the source and the adjacent (connected) unexcited cells comprise the sink,

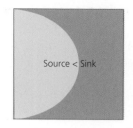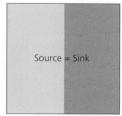

Figure 3.5 Wave curvature and source–sink relationship. The shape of the wave front alters the size of the source and sink.

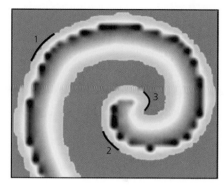

Figure 3.6 Wave curvature along a rotor. Wave curvature is highest at the rotor center (3) (such that propagation fails) and progressively diminishes farther out on the wave front (2 and 1, respectively).

the shape of an activation wave front will influence its source/sink ratio. Convex wave fronts have a smaller source and a larger sink,[3] while flat wave fronts have source–sink balance (Figure 3.5). This means that as wave curvature increases, conduction velocity decreases; with sufficient curvature conduction fails. This is the physiology behind concealed accessory pathways and rotors (Figure 3.6).

Unidirectional block

It is possible for tissue architecture to be arranged such that there is directional asymmetry in source–sink relationships, i.e., with conduction in one direction the source is larger than the sink, while in the opposite direction the source is smaller than the sink. This can occur, for example, with an accessory pathway that

---

[2] While Na^+ and Ca^{++} channels have similar conductance, Na^+ channels activate so much more quickly that they pass more current in a shorter time.

[3] There are a smaller number of excited cells passing current to a larger number of unexcited cells. Picture activation spreading from a focal pacing site (appearing like a growing ring). As the wave spreads, the wave front (source) is a smaller radial distance from the pacing site and the ring of unexcited cells (sink) is at a larger radial distance. Because the circumference increases with radial distance there is always a greater number of sink cells than source cells.

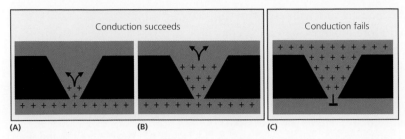

(A)   (B)   (C)

Figure 3.7 Tissue architecture and source–sink mismatch. The physical shape of a fiber can impact the source–sink relationship. A "wedge"-shaped pathway (larger at the top than the bottom) has a different source–sink balance where it connects to the atrial tissue compared with that where it connects to the ventricular tissue. (A) Ventricular muscle (large source) has no difficulty exciting the small accessory pathway fiber at its ventricular insertion site. (B) As the fiber slowly widens the sink is slightly larger than the source, but the balance is sufficient to allow conduction. At the atrial insertion site the fiber has grown wide enough that it provides a sufficiently large source to activate the atrial tissue. (C) With propagation in the opposite direction, the atrial tissue is large enough to excite the wide atrial insertion site of the AP; as the fiber narrows the source is always slightly larger than the sink. Conduction fails at the ventricular insertion site because here the narrow AP is inadequate to depolarize the ventricular muscle to threshold.

is "wedge"-shaped (e.g., the atrial end wider than the ventricular end). Under these conditions, as activation spreads from the ventricle to the narrow end of the pathway the large (ventricular) source is sufficient to depolarize the smaller (pathway) sink. Propagation then spreads along the ever-widening pathway. Because the pathway widens from its ventricular insertion to its atrial insertion, propagation proceeds from narrower portions to wider portions. Thus the sink is larger than the source; if the widening is gradual the sink is only slightly larger than the source and can support conduction. At the accessory pathway–atrial junction the sink is larger still (Figure 3.7A,B; see also Video 3.1) but, if the difference in size is small enough, conduction succeeds. Consider conduction in the opposite direction, from atrium to ventricle. The atrial source is larger than the accessory pathway sink. As propagation proceeds down the progressively narrowing accessory pathway, the source is always larger than the sink. At the accessory pathway–ventricular junction the ratio of accessory pathway cells to adjacent ventricular cells at the narrow end of the pathway is now inadequate to raise the ventricular cells to threshold and conduction fails (Figure 3.7C). This is a concealed pathway (i.e., one that conducts only from ventricle to atrium).[4]

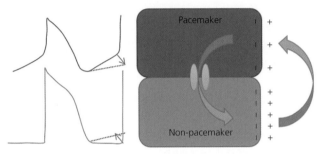

Figure 3.8 Electrotonic current. When a pacemaker cell (top) is electrically connected to a non-pacemaker cell (bottom), current flows down the voltage gradient. This decreases the potential of the pacemaker cell (slowing its rate) and increases the voltage of the non-pacemaker cell (hopefully bringing it to threshold).

Electrotonic interactions

Whenever there is a voltage gradient between two electrically coupled cells there will be current flow between them. This current flow will alter the voltage of both cells (the so-called electrotonic interaction). This current flow has varied effects depending upon the conditions of the two cells. All else being equal (a rare condition), two cells, with different AP morphologies, will be rendered more similar by electrotonic interactions (Figure 3.8).

This has a homogenizing effect on heterogeneous cells when connected in tissue. There is a delicate balance between too little and too much intercellular resistance. A classic example is the interaction between pacemaker and non-pacemaker cells. If there is no connection (or too little connection) intercellular current is insufficient

---

[4] It is called "concealed" because (due to lack of propagation from A to V) there is no pre-excitation and hence the presence of an AP is "concealed" from detection on the EKG.

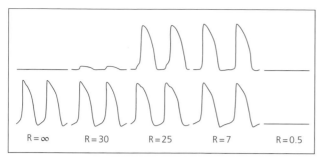

| $R = \infty$ | $R = 30$ | $R = 25$ | $R = 7$ | $R = 0.5$ |

Figure 3.9 Impact of electrotonic currents between a pacemaker and non-pacemaker cell. Shown are the action potentials of a non-pacemaker cell (top) electrically connected with varying resistance (R value in ohms) to a pacemaker cell (bottom). When the two cells are completely disconnected ($R = \infty$) the pacemaker fires at its fastest rate and the non-pacemaker is quiescent. As the resistance decreases, the pacemaker cell slows down (it is using some of its depolarizing current to depolarize the non-pacemaker cell). Once the resistance is low enough, the depolarizing current from the pacemaker cell is diluted too much and neither cell reaches threshold.

to result in propagation from the pacemaker to the non-pacemaker cell. If, on the other hand, the intercellular resistance is too low, so much of the spontaneous depolarizing (pacemaker) current from the pacemaker cell will flow into the non-pacemaker cell that *neither* cell will reach threshold. In fact, within the resistance range that allows propagation without pacemaker suppression, the rate[5] of automaticity is reduced as intercellular resistance is decreased (Figure 3.9).

Anisotropy

Anisotropy refers to direction-dependent conduction velocity. Myocytes are generally longer than they are wide, and gap junctions are not evenly distributed along the cell; they are concentrated at the ends. The result is that

---

[5] Pacemaker rate is related to the time required to depolarize from maximum polarization to threshold; with intercellular current flow some of the inward depolarizing (pacemaking) current leaks to neighbors rather than resulting in depolarization of the pacemaker cell itself. The greater the intercellular flow (lower intercellular resistance), the shallower the slope of phase 4 depolarization and the longer it takes to reach threshold (i.e., the slower the pace rate).

intercellular resistance is lower along the longitudinal than the transverse axis of the tissue. This can influence both conduction velocity and safety factor in complex ways. Lower intercellular resistance will allow current to flow more rapidly between cells (an effect which in isolation would result in increased conduction velocity). However, lower resistance will also increase the size of the sink (by increasing capacitance) and therefore can reduce safety factor and increase the amount of time required to reach threshold (slowing conduction velocity).

Summary

- Excitation requires depolarization to activation threshold.
- Inward current must be sufficient to discharge membrane capacitance.
- Capacitance increases with membrane area; well-connected cells act more like a single large cell.
- Inward current is offset by outward current, and therefore I_{K1} resists depolarization.
- Source–sink balance affects conduction velocity and conduction failure. Source = excited cells. Sink = unexcited cells.
- Safety factor is the amount of current beyond that required to reach activation threshold.
- Due to source–sink balance, conduction velocity (and failure) is dependent upon wave curvature. Spiral waves have sharper curvature closer to the spiral center. At the center, curvature is too small to produce excitation (source–sink mismatch results in block); this creates an area of unexcited cells around which rotation can occur.
- Wedge-shaped accessory pathways can exhibit unidirectional block due to direction-dependent source–sink balance.
- Electrotonic spread of current (between cells) tends to cause homogenization.
- Anisotropy: when conduction velocity is direction-dependent.

4

Arrhythmia mechanisms

The heart is largely made of cells which are passive "drones"; they become excited only in response to excitation of their neighbors. When you ask yourself "what is the mechanism of this rhythm?" you are really asking "what is driving these passive cells?" You can't simply identify a cell as being repetitively activated and conclude that it must be *driving* the rhythm. For example in sinus rhythm every cell would pass the "being repetitively activated" test even though all but the sinus node cells are *being driven*. You could cut off the ventricles (and in fact the atria) and sinus rhythm would persist.

Under various circumstances cardiac tissue is driven by something other than sinus rhythm. This is because some other driver is going faster than the sinus pacemaker cells (either because the sinus node is simply slower than the "other" rhythm or isn't firing at all). What drives these other rhythms? There are several potential mechanisms: automaticity (normal and "abnormal"), triggered firing, and reentry. Of these the vast majority of clinical arrhythmias result from (some form of) reentry. We will review each but concentrate the most on reentry.

It can be useful to think about rhythms in terms of *impulse initiation* and *impulse propagation*. These terms denote the mechanism responsible for creating each beat and the means by which that beat is conducted through the heart, respectively. In some cases the two are intertwined – for instance in reentry, where continuous propagation *is* the mechanism responsible for creating each beat. Rhythms like fibrillation and torsade de pointes combine both impulse initiation and propagation in their mechanisms.

Automaticity

As we've discussed, there are two basic types of cells in the heart, "working-type" and "pacemaker-type" cells. Their difference lies in their behavior during diastole. Working-type cells are the above-mentioned "drones" which wait passively (at rest) until they are activated by intercellular current from their neighbors. Pacemaker cells possess the ability to spontaneously reach threshold and become re-excited on their own (hence the name). Thus it is phase 4 of the action potential where pacemakers and working cells are most different. Pacemaker cells are distributed in multiple locations in the heart. The best-known pacemaker cells are in the sinus node. Best known because under normal conditions these are the cells driving the heart. It is the nature of passive cells that they will be driven by the *fastest* pacemaker. This makes sense, as cells are activated when their neighbors are activated; a faster pacemaker will already have activated cells prior to a slower pacemaker's attempt to do so.[1] Typically atrial, His–Purkinje, and ventricular cells are "working-type," while sinus and atrioventricular (AV) nodal cells are "pacemaker" cells.[2]

---

[1] In fact if the slower pacemakers exhibit "entrance block" such that faster pacemakers do not interact with them, there will be phasic behavior. Intermittently, activation by the slower pacemaker cells will fall between beats generated by the faster pacemaker, thus finding excitable neighbors, and capture/propagate. If the activation wave from the faster cells "penetrates" and depolarizes the slower pacemaker cells, the slower cells will be continuously re-set and there will be no phasic behavior.

[2] There are in fact some latent pacemaker cells in the atria and in the ventricles.

Understanding Clinical Cardiac Electrophysiology: A Conceptually Guided Approach, First Edition. Peter Spector.
© 2016 John Wiley & Sons, Inc. Published 2016 by John Wiley & Sons, Inc.
Companion website: www.wiley.com/go/spector/cardiac_electrophysiology

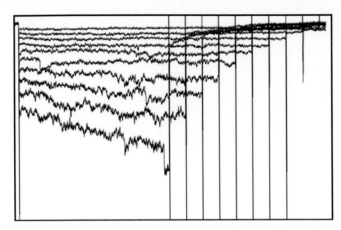
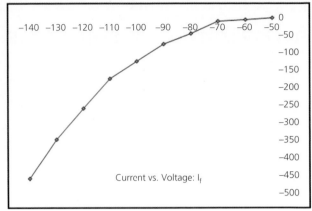

Figure 4.1 **Voltage-dependence of I_f amplitude.** Note that at the typical resting potential of a pacemaker cell there is very little I_f.

Pacemaker cells require two attributes: the **ability to be depolarized** (to threshold) and **intrinsic current** to *cause* that depolarization. As we discussed in Chapter 1, I_{K1} acts as a voltage "clamp" offsetting any inward current and thereby resisting depolarization. Thus a reduced number of I_{K1} channels in a cell is *permissive* of depolarization. With fewer I_{K1} channels, less inward current is required to cause depolarization.

What provides the inward current that causes spontaneous phase 4 depolarization? There are several currents that *can* contribute, but not all are active in all pacemaker cells, as we shall see.

Normal automaticity

Pacemaking currents can be divided into those that contribute to early depolarization (the beginning of phase 4) and those that contribute to late depolarization. Early depolarization is influenced by I_f, as well as deactivation of I_{Kr} and I_{Ks}. Late depolarizing currents include the T-type and L-type calcium currents (I_{CaT} and I_{CaL}), and the sodium–calcium exchange current (NCX).

The "f" in I_f stands for "funny." I_f is called funny because it is a *hyper*polarization-activated channel (Figure 4.1). Deactivation of I_{Kr} and I_{Ks} can also contribute to pacemaking. Pacemaker cells have reduced I_{K1} current, so their resting membrane potential is more depolarized than working-type cells. This is because there is less outward K^+ current to offset inward "leak" currents; resting potential is less negative than the K^+ reversal potential. The balance of currents *immediately following* an action potential, however, favors a membrane potential closer to the K^+ reversal potential. This is because I_{Kr} and I_{Ks} channels transiently remain open

early, after repolarization (which tends to pull the membrane potential towards K^+ reversal potential). As I_{Kr} and I_{Ks} deactivate (close) during early phase 4 the net outward current diminishes, allowing leak (and active pacemaker currents) to depolarize the membrane (Figure 4.2).[3]

As the membrane depolarizes during early phase 4 it reaches the threshold for activation of T-type calcium channels; these contribute to further depolarization (ultimately reaching the activation thresholds for I_{Na} and/or I_{CaL}). There is another *indirect* consequence of T-type calcium current: it triggers release of Ca^{++} from the SR. This indirectly facilitates depolarization because increased Ca^{++} leads to cycling of the Na^+/Ca^{++} exchanger (NCX), producing a net inward current (three Na^+ in exchange for one Ca^{++}).

Abnormal automaticity

Abnormal automaticity refers to the (pathologic) development of spontaneous phase 4 depolarization when cells (which normally rest near K^+ reversal potential) are depolarized. A less negative resting membrane potential can result from a number of causes, but ischemia and stretch are clinically the most common. The depolarizing currents causing this pacemaker activity can vary. In general the more depolarized a cell is the faster its rate of activation. The range of resting potentials at which spontaneous activity occurs is from around –70 mV to –30 mV. Interestingly I_f is inactive at

---

[3] Because this process requires I_{Kr} and I_{Ks} channels that are already open (i.e., requires a *previous* action potential) it is technically not a mechanism for truly *spontaneous* depolarization.

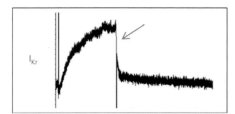 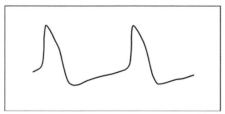

Figure 4.2 Delayed rectifier K⁺ channels and phase 4 depolarization. (Left) The current amplitude of I_{Kr} steadily increases in response to depolarization (recorded during a voltage clamping experiment). Upon repolarization the current abruptly decreases (arrow) due to reduced driving force. It then more slowly diminishes due to channel deactivation. (Right) Action potential of a pacemaker cell. When the cell first repolarizes, K⁺ channels remain open, driving the membrane voltage towards the K⁺ equilibrium potential (like a cell with lots of I_{K1}). Shortly thereafter the delayed rectifiers deactivate, reducing the outward current (diminished voltage clamping effect); the membrane exhibits a "rebound" depolarization.

potentials greater than about –60 mV and hence cannot be responsible for the pacemaker current in this setting. Depolarization can result from any combination of the other currents mentioned above. There is evidence that in some settings I_{Na} or I_{CaL} can contribute as well.

Who cares?

The details of automaticity are not really something that most clinicians need concern themselves with. We discuss it here because it helps to explain things we do concern ourselves with. The general idea that the number of open K⁺ channels influences the ease of pacemaking (depolarization) is helpful to understand. By way of example, why does adenosine cause transient heart block? The answer lies in this very physiology. Under normal circumstances AV node cells (which are latent pacemakers, in part due to low I_{K1} current density) have a relatively depolarized resting membrane potential. However, in the presence of adenosine, the normally closed I_{Kach} channels[4] open, resulting in polarization towards the K⁺ equilibrium potential. Here the amount of resting K⁺ current influences the ease of depolarization (in this case due to cell–cell current *through the AV node*; whereas the impact of K⁺ currents in pacemaker behavior is to reduce depolarization due to intrinsic currents in the pacemaker cell membrane. In the presence of adenosine the membrane is not only hyperpolarized but is "clamped" near potassium equilibrium potential, resisting depolarization and causing transient AV block.

---

[4] The name of the channel and the current it passes are not the same, but it's less confusing to use one name for the current and the channel. I_{KAch} channels are ligand-gated; either adenosine or acetylcholine causes them to open.

Triggered firing

Triggered firing refers to an action potential that arises *as a result of* a preceding action potential. A second action potential arising during repolarization is called an *early after-depolarization* (EAD) while one arising after repolarization is termed a *delayed after-depolarization* (DAD). EADs are felt to be integral to the initiation of torsade de pointes as well as the rapid focal firing that initiates atrial fibrillation;[5] DADs can result from digoxin toxicity.

There is an elegant symmetry between the mechanisms for pulmonary vein (PV) firing and ventricular firing in torsade: both were initially explained by Bela Szabo at the University of Oklahoma.

EADs in torsade

Under normal conditions there is temporal alignment between the duration of membrane depolarization (APD) and the intracellular calcium transient. This alignment can be disrupted. When the APD is increased beyond the calcium transient the membrane is depolarized but intracellular [Ca⁺⁺] is low. This drives the Na⁺/Ca⁺⁺ exchanger "backward"; Ca⁺⁺ "wants" to enter the cell. Current goes where Na⁺ goes, and thus this is a *hyper*polarizing current (which would not cause an after *depolarization*). However, NCX induces an increase in intracellular [Ca⁺⁺] and *that* causes SR Ca⁺⁺ release. SR Ca⁺⁺ release in turn causes the NCX to run "forward," and *this* results in depolarization. If the depolarization is sufficient to reach the threshold for I_{Na} activation, an EAD results (see Chapter 2, Figure 2.15).

---

[5] Typically arising from pulmonary vein (PV) myocytes.

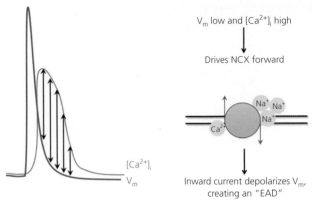

V_m low and [Ca²⁺]ᵢ high

Drives NCX forward

Inward current depolarizes V_m, creating an "EAD"

Figure 4.3 Proposed mechanism of pulmonary vein firing. Shortened APD in the absence of shortened intracellular calcium transient can result in pulmonary vein firing. The combination of membrane polarization and high intracellular calcium drives the NCX forward, creating an inward (depolarizing) current – early after-depolarization.

EADs in PV firing

I_{KAch} is activated in the presence of increased acetylcholine.[6] This directly shortens APD but not the duration of the Ca^{++} transient. Thus membrane voltage is low and intracellular $[Ca^{++}]$ is high, driving the NCX forward (Ca^{++} "wants" to leave the cell and Na^{+} wants to enter). Forward NCX is a depolarizing current; if it causes membrane potential to reach I_{Na} threshold the result is an EAD (Figure 4.3).

Reentry

Reentry is by far the most important arrhythmia mechanism for a clinician to understand.[7] As we will see, premature beats play an important role in initiating reentry (both starting propagation and creating some of the necessary features of the reentry substrate).

Reentry is basically continuous propagation; rather than traversing the tissue and dying out, the wave front perpetually re-excites the tissue.[8] In this way reentry can be thought of as an immortal wave front. Common

---

[6] This is felt to be one of the mechanistic links between ganglionated plexi and AF.

[7] So pay attention.

[8] You can think of normal activation like a wave that travels down a garden hose when you abruptly flick it up and then down. That wave reaches the end of the hose and "extinguishes." Compare this with a hose that loops around such that both ends are connected (after you've started the wave). The wave will reach the "end," propagate to the beginning, and repeatedly re-circulate. Why do you need to connect the ends of the hose *after* you've started the wave?

reentrant arrhythmias include AV nodal reentry, orthodromic reciprocating tachycardia, atrial flutter, scar-mediated atrial and ventricular tachycardias and fibrillation.

Requirements for reentry

If there is to be continuous propagation on a finite surface then cells must be re-excited. Because, once excited, cells are transiently refractory to re-excitation, wave fronts can't simply reverse direction and "back-up."[9] For there to be perpetual propagation the wave front must never encounter (only) unexcitable cells. This means that there must be separate paths for conduction away-from and back-to each site participating in reentry. In short, **reentry requires a circuit** (a continuous loop that "begins" and "ends" in the same place). A circuit is necessary but not sufficient for reentry. There must also be "**unidirectional**" block. This is really an extension of the circuit requirement – a continuous path of excitable cells; in the absence of unidirectional block, activation waves travel both ways around the circuit and collide on the far side (where the wave front is extinguished).[10] Finally, the conduction time around the circuit must be greater than (or equal to) the longest refractory period in the circuit. This, again, is simply an extension of the "continuous path of excitable cells" requirement; if the wave front meets the wave tail (of refractory cells) propagation ceases. This last requirement is often stated as "**wave length must be less than path length**" (see Video 4.1). The wave length is the physical distance between the leading edge of depolarization and the trailing edge of repolarization. The path length is the physical distance around the circuit (Figure 4.4).

Wave length

The wave length is a distance: the distance from the leading edge of excitation to the trailing edge of recovery. Wave length is the product of the refractory period (RP) and the conduction velocity (CV). Thus increasing either CV or RP will increase the wave length. Imagine throwing a ball straight up in the air and seeing how far you can run before the ball falls back to the ground; this

---

[9] Under certain unusual circumstances there can be a phenomenon known as reflection in which "downstream" cells remain excited long enough that "upstream" cells recover from refractoriness and propagation "reflects." This is not clinically relevant physiology.

[10] This is the answer to the question about garden hoses (footnote 8).

is directly analogous to the wave length. If you run faster (conduction velocity) you'll get farther before the ball falls. The time that the ball is in the air is analogous to the action potential duration (refractory period). For any conduction velocity, if it takes longer for the ball to fall you can get farther away before it hits the ground.[11]

Reentry circuits

The actual circuitry that forms the substrate for reentry can vary widely (Figure 4.5; see also Video 4.2), but while the details differ, *all* reentry requires a circuit. The circuit can be structural, i.e., comprised of physically defined paths.[12] Circuits can also be "functional,"

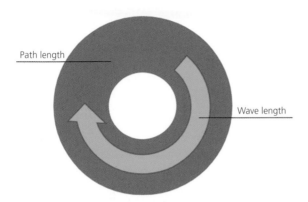

Figure 4.4 Wave length (WL) and path length (PL). The physical distance around a circuit is its path length (gray circle); the distance from the leading edge of excitation to the trailing edge of repolarization is the wave length (green arrow).

meaning the circuit is created by a physiologic failure to conduct rather than a permanent anatomic obstruction to conduction. Functional block can result from transient inexcitability (due to refractoriness) or excitable but unexcited tissue (due to source–sink mismatch). Functional circuits are dynamic; they can change over time and can move through the tissue.

Induction

Regardless of the circuitry, reentry is initiated by unidirectional block enabling a wave to travel in only one direction around the circuit. When the (unidirectional) wave reaches the last portion of the circuit excited before block occurred, these cells must have recovered from refractoriness (wave length < path length).

How does unidirectional block occur? Propagation fails in one limb of a circuit (for any reason). This can result when two paths have different refractory periods; a wave front finds one path excitable but the other blocks due to refractoriness. A difference in refractoriness can occur either because (1) the two paths have different refractory periods (APDs) or because (2) the refractory periods are the same but *out of phase* (i.e., the wave front encounters the two paths at different times relative to the initiation of their respective action potentials) (see Video 4.3).[13] Alternatively both paths may be fully excitable but nonetheless propagation fails in one limb. This

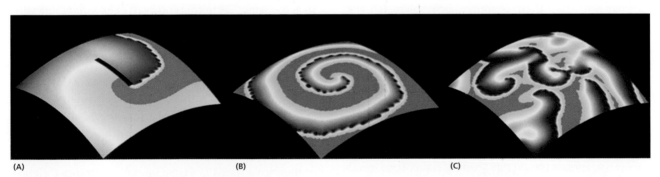

Figure 4.5 Reentry circuits with progressively complex substrate. (A) Structural reentrant circuit – propagation is around an anatomic obstacle. (B) Functional reentrant circuit – in a stable focal rotor, propagation is around excitable but unexcited tissue (due to source–sink mismatch arising from wave curvature). (C) More complex functional reentry – multi-wavelet reentry where substrate is diffuse and dynamic.

---

[11] In reality wave length is complicated: it changes throughout the tissue and over time. Since APD and CV are spatially varied, wave length varies as well.

[12] Examples include: ORT whose circuit is comprised of AVN, ventricular muscle, accessory pathway, and atrial muscle, or VT whose circuit is comprised of scar and surviving channels of myocytes.

[13] A classic example is a PAC delivered close to the atrial insertion site of an accessory pathway. At the time the PAC is delivered both AP and AVN might be refractory (hence block in the AP) but by the time the premature wave propagates through the atrium to the AVN, enough time has elapsed that the node has recovered from refractoriness.

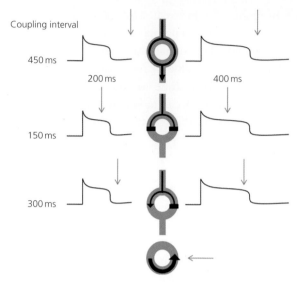

Coupling interval

450 ms

200 ms   400 ms

150 ms

300 ms

Figure 4.6 Programmed stimulation. The idea behind programmed stimulation is to identify a paced coupling interval at which conduction occurs in one limb of a circuit but blocks in the other (unidirectional block), initiating reentry. Here we represent two limbs of a potential circuit (in blue). The refractory periods of the left path is short (200 ms) while that of the right path is long (400 ms). (Top) An extra stimulus at 450 ms falls outside the refractory periods of both paths, thus conducts in both and fuses at the bottom. (Middle) An extra stimulus at 150 ms falls within the refractory periods of both paths and thus blocks in both. (Bottom) An extra stimulus at 300 ms falls outside the refractory period of the left path and hence conducts, but is within the refractory period of the right path, and thus causes unidirectional block and initiates reentry.

can happen when there is source–sink mismatch (i.e., cells are capable of being excited but there is insufficient current to bring them to their activation threshold). Source–sink mismatch can be structural (e.g., a wedge-shaped accessory pathway – see *Unidirectional block* in Chapter 3) or functional (e.g., a curved wave front).

Programmed stimulation

Patients typically come to the EP lab in sinus rhythm, and we need to induce (or attempt to induce) reentry. How do we do it? It is helpful to think about a structural circuit that exists in the heart but is not being used during sinus rhythm.[14] Our job is to "challenge" that circuit (with pacing) such that we create unidirectional block and reentry. I think about a temporal "window" during which a paced beat will conduct in one path but block in the other

(Figure 4.6). We are trying to find that window. If we pace with a coupling interval that is too long, the "extra stimulus" will arrive after both paths have recovered excitability, both will conduct, and the waves will collide on the opposite side of the circuit (no reentry). If we pace with a coupling interval that is too short, the extra stimulus will arrive at both paths before they've recovered from the previous activation and block will occur in both (no reentry). If we pace with a coupling interval that is longer than the RP of one path but shorter than the RP of the other, we'll block in the former and conduct in the latter, initiating reentry (provided WL is < PL). We don't know the refractory periods of the two paths *a priori*. We therefore "scan diastole," i.e., pace at progressively shorter coupling intervals, probing for unidirectional block. In order to be systematic about scanning diastole we want to be sure that the RPs aren't changing over the course of our testing. We know that RP is dynamic, varying with the rate of recent excitation; a phenomenon known as restitution (see Chapter 2). In order to stabilize the RP (so it is the same during each coupling interval tested) we deliver a "conditioning" drive train. This is typically six beats at a fixed paced cycle length. The drive train is then followed by an extra stimulus at a progressively shorter coupling interval for each drive. The larger the discrepancy between the longer and shorter refractory periods the larger the window of inducibility and the more vulnerable the patient is to spontaneous reentry (i.e., due to native premature beats with the "right" coupling interval). The vulnerable window may vary in size (duration) if some condition alters one RP more than the other (e.g., autonomic tone, isoproterenol infusion, or cycle length of the drive train).

It is also possible that our paced beats are not getting to the circuit at the cadence we are delivering them (or not at all). If there is rate-dependent conduction delay between the pace site and the circuit, the coupling interval at the circuit can be longer than at the pace site. Pacing drive trains at faster rates[15] (or from a different site[16]) can improve the ability of the paced beats to arrive

---

[14] i.e., conduction occurs in both directions (no unidirectional block) and collides/fuses at the far side of the circuit, hence there is no reentry in the circuit.

[15] Restitution may decrease the APD of the intervening tissue sufficiently to allow conduction during the fully excitable period, i.e., with no decrease in conduction velocity between the drive train and the extra stimuli.

[16] Different pace sites place different tissue between the paced site and a potential circuit; if the intervening tissue from the second site has better conduction than from the first, induction may be successful from the second even though it failed from the first.

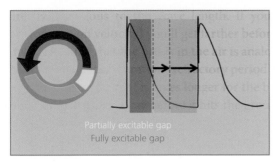

Partially excitable gap
Fully excitable gap

Figure 4.7 The components of the excitable gap. If the wave length of propagation (red arrow) is shorter than the path length of the circuit (blue circle) then there are cells that have recovered from inactivation spanning the distance between the leading edge of excitation (arrow head) and the trailing edge of repolarization (arrow tail). Some of these cells are incompletely recovered (yellow line in circuit); during late repolarization only some of their channels have recovered from inactivation (yellow bar on the action potential tracing). Finally, the remainder of the cells (green line in circuit) have completely recovered from inactivation (green bar on AP tracing) and constitute the fully excitable gap.

at the circuit with the appropriate cadence. This is why we typically perform VT induction studies[17] at two drive cycle lengths and from two sites. A series of extra stimuli (e.g., double or triple extra stimuli) may shorten RP (at the paced site or in the intervening tissue) sufficiently to allow the final extra stimulus to penetrate the circuit.

Factors supporting reentry
- an area of conduction failure (creating a circuit)
- dispersion of refractoriness (increasing the vulnerable window)
- slow conduction (which decreases wave length – maximizing the difference between WL and PL)
- short refractory period (also decreases wave length – maximizing the difference between WL and PL)

Excitable gap
The excitable gap is the physical extent of tissue that separates the trailing edge of repolarization from the leading edge of excitation (it is the difference between wave length and path length) (Figure 4.7). The larger the excitable gap the more stable the reentry. The excitable gap

can be divided into the "fully excitable gap" and the "partially excitable gap." The tissue in the partially excitable gap has recovered some of its ability to be depolarized (some but not all of the Na^+ (or Ca^{++}) channels have recovered from inactivation). A wave front that encroaches upon the relative refractory period will conduct, but with reduced conduction velocity (see Chapter 3); whereas a wave front that encounters the fully excitable gap will conduct at a normal velocity.

Atrial fibrillation: a case study in reentry[18]

In the realm of reentry, fixed anatomic reentry is elegant physiology played out on the simplest possible playing field. Dynamic/functional reentry makes things a lot more interesting and as such is an excellent "classroom" for studying reentry. There is something profound about a tissue which at one moment can support a single, large, organized, propagating wave and at the next exhibits complex multi-wavelet reentry (MWR). What changed? Why are some tissues more susceptible to AF than others?

Spiral waves
Because of source–sink balance, curved waves propagate more slowly than flat waves (see Chapter 3). In fact, as wave curvature increases, the source/sink ratio steadily decreases. Ultimately there is a curvature at which the source is inadequate to activate the sink. At this point there are cells (the sink) that are normal and fully capable of being excited, which are not even refractory, but are nonetheless unexcited. Let's pause here for a moment to consider this. These are cells that behave completely normally when faced with a broad (flat) wave but beyond a certain wave curvature are not excited. So, what happens? Consider the cells that are *not* at the wave end.

These cells have a more favorable source/sink ratio and are able to excite the cells in front of them. In fact, a spiral wave forms because the wave's curvature gets progressively greater toward the spiral center. At the center, the curve's sharpness causes wave break, and produces unexcited cells

---

[17] A means of assessing the risk of sudden cardiac death (rarely used these days).

[18] There are many potential mechanisms for atrial fibrillation, and there is solid evidence for the existence of each of them. The actual mechanism or mechanisms in humans is the subject of much controversy. In this section I will use AF and multi-wavelet reentry interchangeably, but this is almost certainly an oversimplification.

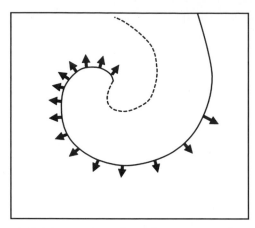

Figure 4.8 Spiral wave. A spiral wave has a progressively greater curve as you progress towards its center. At the center the curvature is so steep that propagation fails due to source–sink mismatch. This creates an area of unexcited cells around which the most central portion of the wave rotates. Interestingly, the majority of the leading edge of activation actually travels in a largely outward (radial) direction (not rotating). As you move outward along the leading edge of the wave front, activation has begun progressively earlier and has therefore propagated farther from the center, giving the appearance of rotation to the entire wave.

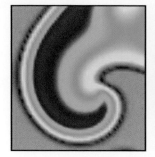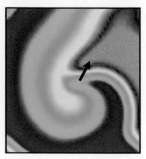

Figure 4.9 Spiral wave meander. When rotor path length (the circumference of the central area of unexcited cells) is less than wave length, the leading edge encounters refractory tissue (its own tail) preventing propagation in a circle. There are excitable cells along the tail (arrow) that allow propagation to continue. As the tail "propagates" (counterclockwise in this example), newly recovered cells become available in its wake and the wave can then rotate as well. The result is a meandering core.

around which rotation can occur. This is a *functional* circuit whose components are formed by "functional" block rather than by a fixed anatomic obstacle. Because curvature decreases (flattens) as we move away from the spiral's center, conduction velocity increases. The curvature is such that at each point along the wave front the conduction velocity causes "rotation" around the ever-increasing circumference at the same cycle length regardless of the distance from the center (Figure 4.8). In reality there is no rotation (except very near the core). Rather there is propagation radially away from the center in which the "trip" start-time is progressively offset as you move circumferentially around the core.

The behavior of a rotor is dependent upon the balance between wave length and path length at the rotor core. We've already discussed the restriction that wave length must be less than path length (or collision causes the wave to extinguish). What determines the wave length and the path length in a functional circuit? The minimum curvature is a function of tissue excitability (due to its influence on sink size) and action potential duration (due to its influence on source size). The curvature will determine how sharply the wave can turn and in part sets the "circumference" of rotation (i.e., the path length). The curvature plus the other factors that influence source and sink (see Chapter 3) will determine conduction

velocity; CV and APD will determine the wave length. So what happens if the wave length is longer than the circumference set by the minimum "turning radius"? Unlike the case with fixed anatomic reentry, this circuit is dynamic. If the wave front travels around the minimum curvature only to encounter its refractory tail it simply propagates along that tail until it reaches excitable cells (Figure 4.9). Therefore, while wave length cannot be longer than path length, the path length can expand to accommodate this restriction; the circuit "core" changes from a circle (or point) to a line.

A quick look at the preceding paragraph makes clear that the factors which determine the circuit are almost all functional, having much to do with how the tissue was recently activated. Thus it should not be surprising that because these things can vary in an ongoing fashion, waves can meander around the tissue.

What initiates a rotor in the first place? In order for a rotor to form there must be a "free wave end." By this we mean a wave front that has at least one end that *isn't* on the outer boundary of the tissue. Typically, waves will have both ends on the tissue's edge (Figure 4.10A) or will have no wave ends (i.e., a circular wave – Figure 4.10B). The free wave end requirement relates to the "circuit requirement" story of reentry. As we've discussed, reentry is continuous propagation; for continuous propagation to occur (on a finite tissue) the wave front must perpetually encounter *excitable tissue*. Unless there is a circuit the physical/spatial relationship between the leading edge of excitation and the supply of excitable cells is such that propagation "uses up" all the excitable cells. Try to

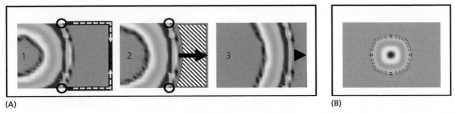

Figure 4.10 Wave ends, boundaries, and fuel supply. (A) (1) If the two ends of a wave (circles) are on the same boundary (red line), as the wave propagates, the ends will approach each other along the boundary (yellow arrows). (2) The supply of excitable cells (striped area) is bounded by the edge of the tissue and the wave front. (3) The area of excitable cells progressively diminishes until there are no more excitable cells and propagation ceases. (B) Focal excitation initiates a concentric wave which has a continuous wave front and hence no ends. As the wave front reaches the boundary it will split, producing waves which have both ends on the same boundary. Once again the supply of excitable cells steadily diminishes.

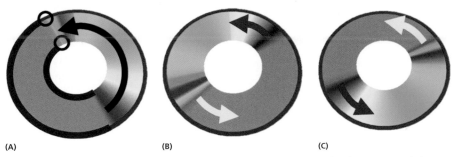

Figure 4.11 Wave ends on separate boundaries creates a circuit. (A) When the two ends of a wave (circles) are on separate boundaries (red lines) the supply of excitable cells (gray) is bounded by the wave front, the two boundaries, *and the wave tail.* (B) The result is that the area of excitable cells *never changes* because the wave tail (blue arrow) is moving at the same rate and in the same direction (counterclockwise in this example) as the wave front (yellow arrow). (C) This defines a circuit and allows for perpetual propagation.

imagine propagation using a "fuel" and "fire" analogy: the leading edge of excitation is the fire, and to continue burning it requires a continuous supply of fuel (excitable cells). Unlike real fuel, cardiac cells, once recovered from refractoriness, can become fuel again. So as a wave front traverses excitable tissue it leaves a wake of refractory cells and farther behind a tail of recovered/excitable cells. In order for propagation to perpetuate, the leading edge must come into physical contact with the line of re-excitable cells behind the wave tail. A circuit is (by definition) a spatial relationship that places the wave front in contact with *this* tail.[19] Consider an activation wave traversing tissue *without* a circuit (Figure 4.10). In this case both wave ends are on the same boundary, and as propagation progresses the supply of excitable cells is

consumed; eventually the two wave ends meet and propagation ceases.

Wave break creates the substrate for reentry – two wave ends on separate boundaries (Figure 4.11). Reentry requires more than simply the existence of a circuit, there must be unidirectional block and WL < PL. *Wave break*, in this case, creates the circuit and *is the unidirectional block.* The path length is the inner circumference of rotation.

The initiation of a rotor requires wave break (which creates a free wave end); wave break occurs due to structural or functional block. Heterogeneity of APD (and hence refractoriness) enhances the likelihood of wave break. Rapid firing (due to pacing or spontaneous ectopy) sets the stage for one wave to collide (in some places but not others) with the tail of the prior wave, initiating wave break and rotation. The rotor can be spatially stable (if the wave length is less than the inner circumference of rotation) or can meander (if the wave length is longer than the inner circumference). Finally, the rotor not only has a core around which rotation occurs but also a spiral-shaped wave front emanating

---

[19] Don't confuse this "wave-front-meets-tail" with the wave front meeting the unexcitable tail (which leads to an extinguished wave). In this case we are speaking specifically about the line of cells *behind* the refractory tail which have just recovered (or any cells farther from the tail).

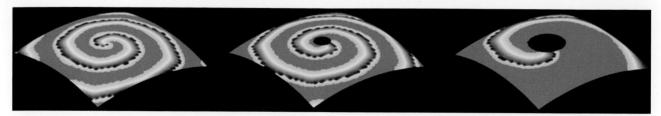

Figure 4.12 Focal ablation does not terminate reentry. Reentry can perpetuate as long as there is an uninterrupted circuit. Therefore focal ablation at the center of a rotor *does not* result in termination (no matter how large the lesion). Instead the functional circuit (rotor) is transformed into a structural circuit (around the focal ablation).

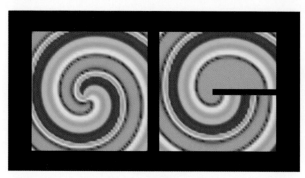

Figure 4.13 Termination requires circuit transection. By creating a linear lesion from the outer boundary (tissue edge) to the inner boundary (the rotor core) we produce a *single* boundary. Now both wave ends are on the same boundary and the excitable cells will inevitably be consumed, extinguishing propagation.

from that core. *That* wave front can also break, spawning new rotors and leading to multi-wavelet reentry.

Once reentry starts, how does it stop? The answer lies in the circuit requirement for reentry: interrupt the circuit, and the supply of excitable cells eventually runs out and reentry terminates. *Anything* that results in circuit interruption will cause termination of reentry. Clinically that could mean spontaneous ectopy resulting in bidirectional conduction, antiarrhythmic medication causing wave length to increase beyond path length, or ablation physically interrupting a circuit.

An important implication of the circuit requirement is that focal ablation at the center of a rotor *will not* directly cause termination (Figure 4.12; see also Video 4.4).[20] Termination of a rotor requires the same thing as termination of any reentrant rhythm – interruption of its circuit. From an ablation perspective this means linear ablation leading from the rotor core to the tissue edge; this turns a circuit (a loop around func-

 tional block) into a U-shaped path (a peninsula created by the ablation) around which rotation cannot occur (Figure 4.13; see also Video 4.5).

How does multi-wavelet reentry ever *spontaneously* terminate? To answer this question let's talk about how any rotor terminates. Something must cause circuit interruption. That "something" is sufficient meander of the core such that it collides with the tissue edge (Figure 4.14; see also Video 4.6). At this point the two ends of the rotor's wave front are on the same boundary (the tissue edge) so all excitable cells will be consumed. This can occur for example if the "untethered"[21] wave end collides with a refractory wave tail and travels along it to the tissue's edge. In multi-wavelet reentry, multiple waves simultaneously co-exist; when each of these collides with a boundary and is interrupted, no waves exist and MWR terminates.

The mass hypothesis

What makes one heart more prone to MWR than another? First, a higher likelihood of wave break leading to *initiation* (e.g., spontaneous focal firing and refractory heterogeneity). Second, a lower likelihood of *termination* (i.e., decreased probability of circuit core collision[22]). Let's address the second issue – likelihood of termination. It seems logical that in larger tissues (more precisely, tissues with a larger area) there is a lower likelihood of core collision with a boundary. Tissues of different shapes have a different ratio of boundary length (total edge length) to tissue area. As area gets larger and boundary length gets smaller the likelihood of collision decreases; this increases the stability of MWR. In addition, a shorter wave length allows a greater number of waves

---

[20] In fact focal ablation may simply convert a functional circuit into a structural circuit.

[21] We use the term "free wave end" or "untethered wave end" to describe a wave end that is not attached to the tissue edge or other physical boundary.
[22] With an outer boundary.

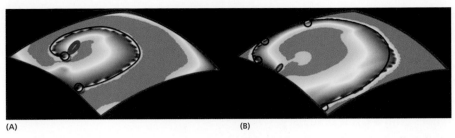

Figure 4.14 Spontaneous rotor termination. (A) wave ends are on different boundaries, the outer (red) and inner/functional boundary (blue); reentry persists as long as there is a circuit. (B) When the rotor core collides with the outer boundary there is only one boundary (all red), so all wave ends are on the same boundary; the circuit no longer exists, resulting in inevitable termination.

to co-exist per unit area of tissue. With a larger number of waves the probability that *all* will collide and annihilate is lower. This basic formulation was hypothesized nearly a hundred years ago by Dr. Garrey. He studied fibrillation in superfused tissue preparations by touching AC current to the tissue and watching it physically wriggle (he made no electrical recordings). He noted that the propensity to fibrillate was directly proportional to tissue area. He wondered whether the *shape* of the tissue mattered. Further studies indicated that in two tissues with the same area but different shapes, the skinnier tissue was less able to support fibrillation. This boils down to a higher area-to-boundary-length ratio being pro-fibrillatory. The mass hypothesis helps to explain the progressive nature of AF. Atrial fibrillation leads to dilation (increased area) but not increased boundary length, thereby increasing the area/boundary-length ratio. It also results in interstitial fibrosis and altered expression of gap junctions (decreasing conduction velocity) as well as altered expression of ion channels (shortening action potential durations). These changes produce a shorter wave length; all are pro-fibrillatory alterations.

We can better understand AF therapies in the context of the mass hypothesis: treatments either increase wave length (antiarrhythmic drugs and ablation of ganglionated plexi) or increase boundary length (ablation).

Summary

- **Automaticity:** phase 4 depolarization requires inward current and lack of the voltage "clamping" effect of I_{K1}.

- Pacemaker currents:
  - **Early:** I "funny" (I_f) – hyperpolarization-activated inward current; deactivation of I_{Kr} and I_{Ks}.
  - **Late:** T-type and L-type calcium currents and sodium–calcium exchange current.
- **Abnormal automaticity:** membrane depolarization can lead to spontaneous phase 4 depolarization.
- **Triggered firing:**
  - Ventricle: long action potential duration and normal calcium transient leads to high membrane voltage and low intracellular [Ca^{++}]; this leads to "backward" sodium–calcium exchange current; this causes SR calcium release; which causes forward sodium–calcium exchange current (inward current) and early after-depolarizations (EADs).
  - Pulmonary vein: acetylcholine causes shortened APD but normal calcium transient; low membrane voltage and high intracellular [Ca^{++}] causes forward sodium–calcium exchange current (inward current) and EADs.
- **Reentry:** requires a closed circuit, unidirectional block, and wave length (WL) < path length (PL).
- **Factors supporting reentry:** a circuit, dispersion of refractoriness, slow conduction velocity, and short refractory period.
- **Excitable gap:** the time/distance between recovery from inactivation and re-excitation.
- **Wave length** = conduction velocity × refractory period.
- **Atrial fibrillation:**
  - Spiral waves: curvature-dependent conduction velocity; at the sharpest curvature source–sink mismatch causes conduction failure and unexcited cells around which rotation can occur.
  - If WL < PL, the wave traverses along its refractory tail until it meets recovered tissue and then rotates – causing meander.

- Wave break along the spiral arm can cause new spiral formation and multi-wavelet reentry (MWR).
- Initiation: when the leading edge of a wave encounters refractory tissue (non-uniform) the result is wave break and rotation.
- Termination: circuit interruption occurs when a circuit core collides with a tissue boundary. When all circuits are interrupted MWR terminates.
- Factors that decrease the probability of core collisions increase fibrillogenicity: increased tissue area, decreased boundary length, decreased wave length (allowing more waves) – mass hypothesis of AF.

5

Anatomy for electrophysiologists

Anatomy is anatomy, but electrophysiologists think about it from a slightly different perspective than most. The standard approach to cardiac anatomy (the course you took in medical school) is like the song "the atria bone is connected to the ventricle bone"; we learn cardiac anatomy from a plumbing perspective. In EP we are less concerned with how blood flows and more concerned with (1) how electricity flows and (2) what things are spatially adjacent but *not* electrically connected. The importance of the former to an electrophysiologist is obvious. The issue with the latter is this: electric current generates a potential field detectable at a distance. Thus it is not only on the ventricle that we can "see" a ventricular electrogram. The potential field generated by local ventricular depolarization is large enough that an electrode in a nearby portion of the atrium can record a significant electrogram. Therefore the onus is on us to determine which of our signals are "near-field" (local activation) and which are "far-field." There are characteristics of the electrogram that help to make this distinction (see Chapter 8), but a major consideration is "what electrically active structures are nearby."

A significant challenge for electrophysiologists is the fact that we can't see the heart; we don't open the chest. Instead we use many indirect means of detecting cardiac anatomy to deduce its structure. We'll go through some of the tools shortly, but the gist of how we approach cardiac anatomy is to form a mental map of the heart's 3D anatomy; we then use what we *can* see to "register" ourselves with that mental map. Think about navigating from your bed at night in the dark. You sit up and feel for your bedside table and then, knowing where you are and combining that with a mental picture of your bedroom, you can walk to the bathroom.

The 3D anatomy of the heart is surprisingly complex; it's a lot to try to keep in your head. Truly learning anatomy is a long-term project. I have found it extremely helpful to focus intensely on one region at a time. Whenever I'm doing a case that involves a certain aspect of anatomy I try to deeply digest that region. How do you learn the anatomy in the first place? Diagrams and pictures are great, but there is no substitute for 3D viewing and the ability to spin the heart around and look at it from many different angles. It can be extremely helpful to go to your hospital's pathology department and dissect hearts with a pathologist. A close second to this is modern CT and MRI viewers that allow you to make 3D reconstructions of the whole heart. You can rotate them and slice through them over and over. Switching between rotating the 3D heart and "scanning through" the 2D slices can be quite helpful as well. My advice is to do this for *every* case in which you have pre-procedural 3D imaging.

Some of the currently available mapping systems allow you to import 3D reconstructions. The advantage of these systems is that you can select individual components of the anatomy – e.g., right atrium (RA) or left atrium (LA) – and show or hide them. This is a great way to appreciate the relationship between structures.

Sadly you will find, as you read and talk to your colleagues, that the terminology used by electrophysiologists can be ambiguous. For example (given the tilt of the heart in the chest) the terms superior and anterior are frequently used interchangeably, as are inferior and posterior. In the ventricle it is clear what is meant when one says apical or basal; there are no universally accepted correlates for those same directions when talking about atrial anatomy. The terms annular and "anti-annular" work – though I don't think I've ever

Understanding Clinical Cardiac Electrophysiology: A Conceptually Guided Approach, First Edition. Peter Spector.
© 2016 John Wiley & Sons, Inc. Published 2016 by John Wiley & Sons, Inc.
Companion website: www.wiley.com/go/spector/cardiac_electrophysiology

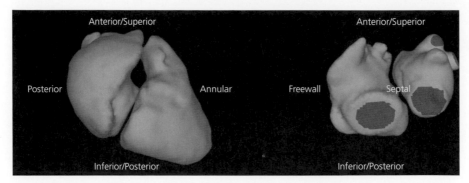

Figure 5.1 Conventional terminology for atrial anatomy. When conventional terminology is applied to atrial anatomy it is somewhat ambiguous. Anterior and superior are referred to interchangeably as are inferior and posterior. What is referred to as basal and apical in the ventricles is posterior and annular in the atria.

heard anyone say anti-annular. Instead, the anti-annular direction is often called posterior whereas the floor is called inferior. Septal and freewall are pretty self-explanatory, although this gets somewhat complicated in the right ventricular (RV) outflow tract as you head "out of the heart" towards the pulmonary artery (PA).

We will use the following conventions (Figure 5.1): atrial "directions" are posterior vs. annular, anterior/superior vs. inferior/posterior, and septal vs. freewall; ventricular directions are anterior vs. posterior/inferior, septal vs. freewall, and basal vs. apical.

A tour of cardiac anatomy

Right atrium

The superior vena cava (SVC) enters the superior aspect of the RA (Figure 5.2). Annular to the SVC (and towards the left) is the ascending aorta. As you enter the heart the annular direction takes you straight into the right atrial appendage (RAA). Immediately between the SVC orifice and the RAA is Bachmann's bundle, a group of parallel fibers that provide rapid conduction from RA (sinus node) to LA. Posterior to the RA (as you enter via the SVC ostium) is the right superior pulmonary vein (RSPV). It is common to see far-field RSPV potentials from the posterior–superior RA (Figure 5.3).

How can you distinguish far-field from near-field in the posterior RA?

In addition to electrogram characteristics (see Chapter 8) you can examine activation sequence. If activation is truly from the right it will spread away from the posterior

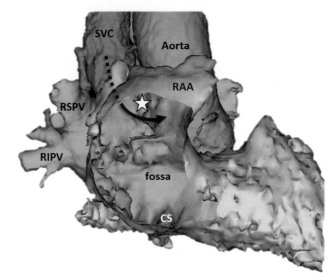

Figure 5.2 Right atrium. Traveling in the annular direction as you enter the RA from the SVC (arrow), you pass Bachmann's bundle (star) and enter the right atrial appendage. CS, coronary sinus; RIPV, right inferior pulmonary vein.

wall (radially) including towards the septum/Bachmann's bundle area. On the other hand, if activation is arising from the RSPV, then RA activation will be in the opposite direction, from septum/Bachmann's bundle towards the posterior RA.

Laterally (freewall) in the RA there is a junction between a region of trabeculated and smooth RA (Figure 5.4). This junction is called the crista terminalis (endocardially) and the sulcus terminalis (epicardially). The sulcus is where the sinus node sits. The crista is a *potential* barrier to conduction; not infrequently one sees "double potentials" along the crista; one potential from its posterior aspect and one from its annular aspect. The crista is a common site for focal atrial tachycardias.

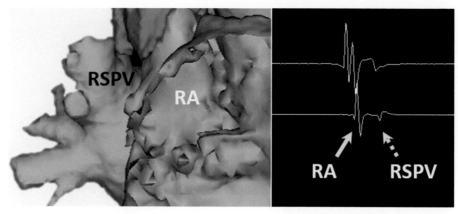

Figure 5.3 Posterior RA vs. right superior pulmonary vein. Because the RSPV is adjacent to the posterior RA one can often record electrograms from one with a catheter in the other. Understanding which structures are sufficiently close to allow for such "far-field" recording is critical to performing EP safely and effectively.

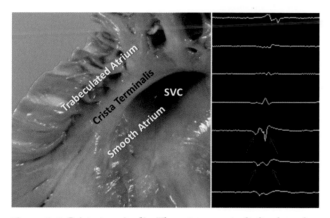

Figure 5.4 Crista terminalis. The crista terminalis lies lateral to the entrance of the SVC into the RA. The crista can act as an obstacle to conduction from the trabeculated to the smooth RA, resulting in double potentials along the lateral RA.

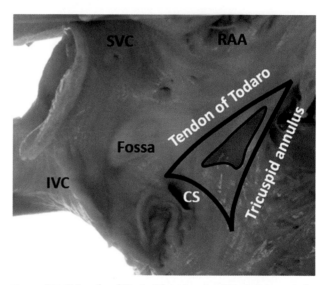

Figure 5.5 Triangle of Koch. The triangle of Koch is bounded posteriorly by the tendon of Todaro, inferiorly by the coronary sinus, and annularly by the tricuspid annulus. The compact AV node (shown in red) sits in the triangle.

There is a continuous connection from Bachmann's bundle into the crista terminalis, becoming the Eustachian ridge at the lateral inferior aspect of the RA, and becoming the tendon of Todaro (TT) at the septal inferior aspect of the RA. The tendon leads into the cartilaginous ring supporting the tricuspid valve at the peak of the triangle of Koch (Figure 5.5) (see below).

As you proceed inferiorly along the septal side of the RA from the RA–SVC junction you cross over the limbus, a thick unyielding fibrous structure that marks the superior entrance to the fossa ovalis. The limbus (as we'll see) causes a trans-septal needle to deviate from a leftward position as it is pulled down the SVC, moving it rightward as it crosses over the limbus and resulting in a marked leftward "jump" as it falls into the fossa (Figure 5.6; see also Video 5.1).

Sub-Eustachian isthmus

If you enter the RA inferiorly (retrograde from the RV) you cross the tricuspid annulus (TA) and enter the sub-Eustachian (or cavo-tricuspid) isthmus. The "isthmus" plays an important role in EP, as it is frequently the target for ablation in patients with "typical" atrial flutter. The isthmus is partially bounded by the TA, the coronary sinus (CS), and the Eustachian ridge (Figure 5.7). Along its lateral aspect there is no specific demarcation as it "opens up" to the RA freewall. The isthmus can vary quite a bit. Often there are thick trabeculae that extend in from the freewall. It can be very narrow or wide and

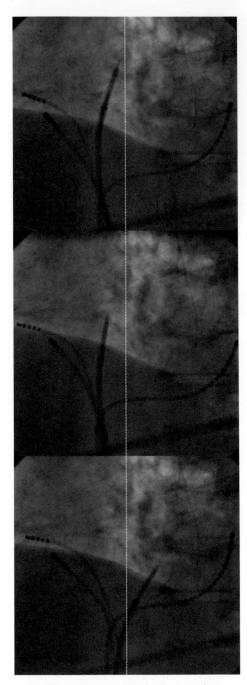

Figure 5.6 Needle passing over the limbus. As the trans-septal needle is pulled down from the SVC, it is forced rightward (left side of image) as it crosses over the limbus. Beneath the limbus it abruptly shifts leftward (right side of image) into the fossa ovalis.

is often shaped like a pouch. These are all features that impact ablation, and hence it is often wise to do a little reconnaissance prior to ablating.[1] The ridge acts as a functional obstacle to conduction. As a result a "CTI line"[2] need not actually extend all the way from the TA to the IVC; it can stop at the ridge.

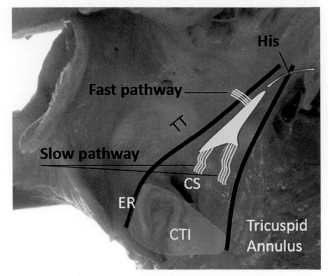

Figure 5.7 Triangle of Koch and cavo-tricuspid isthmus. The tendon of Todaro (TT) and the tricuspid annulus (TA) meet at the top of the triangle of Koch. This is where the His bundle extends from the top of the compact AV node. The fast pathway fibers extend over the tendon superiorly; slow pathway fibers extend from the inferior portion of the node to the roof of the coronary sinus (CS). The tendon of Todaro continues laterally as the Eustachian ridge (ER). The cavo-tricuspid isthmus (CTI) spans between the ER and the TA.

Triangle of Koch

The septal annular aspect of the RA is a major focus in EP. This is where the AV node (AVN), fast and slow pathways (FP/SP), and the beginnings of the His are found. The triangle of Koch is the center of attention (Figure 5.7). The triangle is demarcated by the TA, the CS os, and the TT. The AVN sits in the center of the triangle with the fast pathway fibers exiting the triangle by crossing the TT superiorly, typically about one-third of the way from the top (His recording region) to the bottom (CS os). The slow pathway is often much more complex than the fast pathway; there can be many SPs. There is a rightward SP that can be found anywhere from the TA to the CS os. There are also, often, leftward extensions of the SP inserting into the roof of the CS, at times as far laterally as 4:00–5:00 on the mitral annulus (MA).[3]

---

[1] Moving your catheter along the planned path of ablation to see if there is a pouch and assess the "reach" (distance from ridge to TA). You can also examine the electrogram voltage, which correlates with thickness/trabeculae.

[2] Ablation line crossing the "cavo-tricuspid isthmus."

[3] Positions along the MA are often referred to as if the MA were a clock face viewed from below in the LAO projection (see Chapter 6, *LAO*): anterior = 12:00, posterior = 6:00, freewall = 3:00, septal = 9:00.

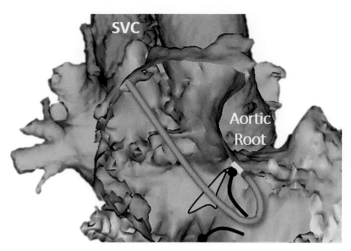 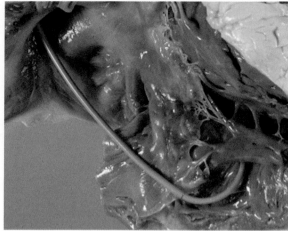

Figure 5.8 **His bundle, aortic root, and tricuspid annulus.** The His bundle extends from the superior aspect of the AV node (green) and penetrates through the cartilaginous ring of the tricuspid valve annulus (black dots). As a result one can often ablate anteroseptal accessory pathways from beneath the tricuspid leaflet where the endocardial AP can be heated, while the penetrating bundle is relatively protected by the valve ring. It is important to note that radiofrequency (RF) ablation at this site will likely result in permanent right bundle branch block.

Antero-annular RA

The His bundle can be recorded at the top of the triangle of Koch. Above (superior) sits the root of the aorta (Figure 5.8). As a result one can often record a His potential from the root of the aorta. This apposition of aorta with RAA/superior annular RA also means that when sticking a needle through that part of the RA one could enter the aorta. This apposition can be capitalized upon; some epicardial focal right atrial tachycardias can be ablated from the root of the aorta (as can some VTs).

There is another relatively import anatomical "tidbit." At the anteroseptal RV the His bundle dives through the cartilaginous valve ring (the "penetrating bundle"). The His is relatively thermally protected in this location. Using the SVC approach, a catheter placed beneath the tricuspid valve and pulled can target anteroseptal accessory pathways with modest protection of normal AV conduction (Figure 5.8). Not only is the His within the cartilage at this point (and hence somewhat protected from heating) but with the catheter tucked under the valve it is much less likely to slide and deliver energy to other vulnerable sites (e.g., FP, compact node).

Right ventricle

The RV actually has a fairly complex shape (Figure 5.9). There is an RV inflow (TA region) and an RV outflow (RVOT). The PA and aorta twist across each other anterior to the heart (such that at a sufficiently superior level the aorta is posterior and *to-the-right-of* the PA. The RVOT and LVOT therefore have a changing degree of "rotation," with the RVOT transitioning from rightward-and-in-front-of the LVOT to become next-to-and-leftward-of the LVOT.

One thing that we must bear in mind when delivering RF is "what's on the other side of this tissue." An example of the significance of this question is the difference in consequence of a perforating steam pop[4] in a septal region (i.e., one that separates one chamber from another) vs. in a freewall region (i.e., one where there is pericardium opposite the RF site). Also, there are places in the apical aspect of the RAA or the posterior aspect of the RVOT where one is very close to the right coronary artery and should hence be cautious when burning.

Left atrium – pulmonary vein

The LA comes in many shapes and sizes. In general there are four pulmonary veins (right and left, each with an upper and lower). Frequently the upper and lower

---

[4] During delivery of RF (or any form of ablation that employs heating) heating the tissue beneath the surface to greater than 100 °C can result in the water in the tissue turning to steam, expanding, and dissecting through the tissue to relieve that pressure. This is called a steam pop. A steam pop that vents to the endocardial surface increases the risk of thrombus formation; one that vents to both sides causes a perforation.

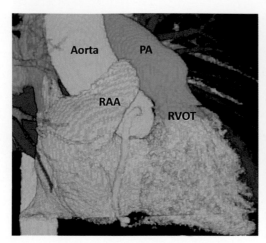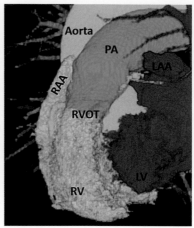

Figure 5.9 **Right ventricle.** The RV as viewed from the RAO (right) and LAO (left) projections.

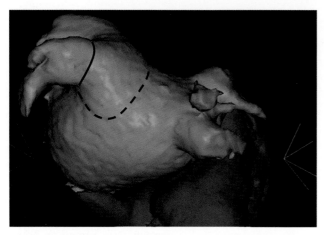

Figure 5.10 **Pulmonary veins.** The electrical junction between PV and LA is at the PV–antrum junction (solid line). The antrum meets the LA at the antrum–LA junction (dashed line). There is no electrical signature of the antrum–LA junction.

veins are separate as they enter the atrium. In some cases the two fuse prior to entering the atrium, forming a so-called "common os." In either case the vein ostia frequently enter into an antrum (a more or less pronounced antechamber) and then into the LA proper. There are two junctions between the PV and LA; the PV–antrum junction and the antrum–LA junction (Figure 5.10). The PV–antrum is the electrical junction between PV and LA. There are discontinuities in conduction between these two tissues. There are typically double potentials[5] along this junction, reflecting either true local disconnection or slowed conduction (Figure 5.11). Atrial muscle extends a small distance

---

[5] See Chapter 8.

into the pulmonary veins. This "sleeve" of myocytes is rarely connected to the atrial tissue along its entire circumference. There are discrete (electrical) connections from PV to LA, with conduction to the remainder of the PV tissue spreading parallel to the junction once it has entered the PV (Figure 5.11). These connections can be along a large or small percentage of the circumference, and there can be one or more connections. Typically the musculature only travels ~1 cm into the PV.

The roof of the LA is not horizontal; the RSPV and LSPV do not enter the LA at the same height (Figure 5.10). Very often the roof slants downwards as you travel from the left to the right. This is a common source of frustration for the unwitting fellow. If you put "clockwise" torque on the catheter while at the os of the LSPV (in an attempt to move it to the RSPV) without first pulling down, torque builds up, as the roof impedes rotation, and ultimately the catheter flies around, markedly overshooting the RSPV. Also the upper and lower PVs are not lined up vertically: the superior veins are more annular than the inferior veins.

Left atrium

If you look at a CT scan of the LA you'll often notice a prominent "dent" in its superior annular aspect (Figure 5.12). This is where the non-coronary and left coronary aortic cusps lie. The size and shape of the left atrial appendage (LAA) is extremely variable. It can take off from near the roof of the LA or much closer to

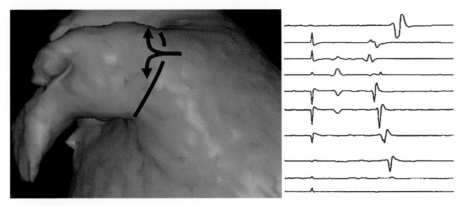

Figure 5.11 PV–antrum junction. There is a discrete electrical connection between the PV and the LA at the PV–antrum junction (left). One can see a pacing artifact followed by early far-field potentials from the LA and, later, near-field potentials within the PV (right). The site of PV–LA connection can be identified by the earliest PV potential provided conduction is *into* the vein.

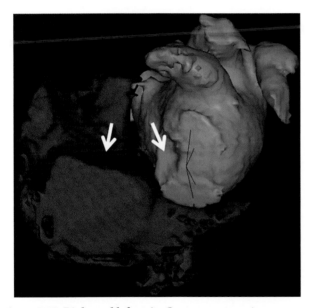

Figure 5.12 Right and left atria. One can see prominent "dents" in the atria where they meet the root of the aorta.

the floor. It can be short or long, straight or zigzagged.[6] There is a "ridge" that separates the left pulmonary veins and the LAA. The ridge can be like a mesa (large and flat), but more often it is a narrow lip. This markedly influences the ability to achieve adequate catheter tissue contact when performing an LPV-encircling ablation. Along the epicardial aspect of this ridge (between the LSPV and LAA) runs the ligament of

Marshall (LOM). The LOM is a fibrous band that is a vestige of the *in utero* left SVC which becomes the (often vestigial) vein of Marshall (and the associated ligament of Marshall). This has been found to cause focal firing that triggers AF in some patients. It can also (rarely) provide an epicardial electrical connection between the LPVs and the CS musculature.[7]

The esophagus lies posterior to the LA. It is not adhered to the heart and can thus move relative to the heart. The two structures are very close to each other, such that energy delivered in the posterior LA can heat the esophagus. In the worst-case scenario this can lead to an atrial–esophageal fistula (though very rare, often a fatal complication). The practice in our lab is to assume that the esophagus is anywhere *it could possibly be* and deliver energy accordingly (we use lower power for shorter durations). The esophagus cannot cross the PVs and hence cannot be annular to the PVs. The esophagus is not a straight vertical tube; it can wrap around the LA, touching it from fairly annular along the roof to various extents along the floor.

Coronary sinus

The coronary sinus (CS) is a vein that drains into the RA (remember that the CS os defines the base of the triangle of Koch). It runs parallel to the mitral annulus (Figure 5.13).[8] As you proceed ("upstream") into the

---

[6] Electrophysiologists have taken to studying the various LAA shapes in the era of LAA closure devices. The location of the take-off is important for those attempting to deliver a left mitral isthmus (LMI) ablation line.

[7] Allowing propagation between the two without activating the atrial tissue in between.

[8] The ostium of the CS can be partially obstructed by the Thebesian valve.

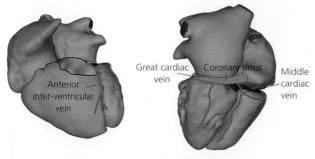

Figure 5.13 Coronary sinus and cardiac veins. The coronary sinus runs along the mitral annulus (frequently overlying the atrium not the ventricle).

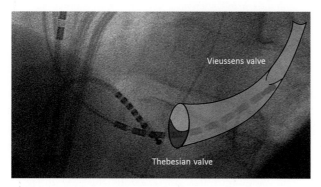

Figure 5.14 Valves of the coronary sinus. The entrance of the CS can sometimes be partially obstructed by the Thebesian valve. The coronary sinus is separated from the great cardiac vein by the Vieussens valve.

CS from the RA at about 4:00 you encounter the Vieussens valve (Figure 5.14).[9] This valve separates the CS proper from the great cardiac vein (GCV). The GCV wraps all the way around the annulus, reaching the superior septal aspect of the MA. At this point it turns and runs along the interventricular septum as the anterior interventricular vein. There are a variable number of ventricular venous branches off of the CS/GCV.[10] The CS has electrically active musculature and is connected to both the right and left atria. Connections exist at the CS os (RA) and along the roof of the CS up to the valve/GCV (LA). These electrical connections can play a prominent role

---

[9] It is not uncommon to get your catheter stuck between the valve and the CS wall, preventing placement of the catheter into the great cardiac vein. If you anticipate encountering the valve (and where), you can simply back up a little and redirect the tip, then re-advance until you cross into the GCV.

[10] These can be quite useful for pacing the left ventricle without actually entering the LV.

in arrhythmias. The leftward extensions of the slow AV nodal pathway often insert into the CS musculature along the roof of the CS. The musculature can extend down into the middle cardiac vein (MCV). This vein runs along the inferior interventricular septum. Under some pathologic conditions the MCV musculature can electrically connect to the underlying LV, creating an accessory AV pathway (AP). These pathways thus have complex atrial connections; the MCV connects to the CS musculature and from there extensively connects to both the left and right atria. "Earliest A" (see *Mapping accessory pathways,* Chapter 9) in this case does *not* truly reflect the upper end of the AP; the earliest CS activation indicates a discrete upper end of the AP.

The coronary sinus plays a prominent role in clinical EP for anatomic reasons as well. It is aligned parallel to the mitral annulus and thus allows a catheter to record from both the left atrium and ventricle. Because the CS is a tubular structure, a catheter placed in the CS is physically stable (i.e., less likely to spontaneously move). Its position along the annulus makes it a very useful guide for diagnosis, mapping, and ablation, particularly of left-sided APs. We will see at length, later, that by placing a multi-electrode catheter in the CS we have several spatially stable electrograms which aid in interpretation of activation sequence. While the CS is parallel to the MA it is very often located over the *atrium* near the MA rather than on the annulus itself; hence ventricular signals are often "more far-field" than the atrial or CS signals.

Left ventricle

The LV has two very prominent anatomic features – the anterior and posterior papillary muscles which connect, via the chordal apparatus, to the mitral valve. These can impede smooth catheter manipulation in the area. There are two ways to put a catheter into the LV: across the interatrial septum then through the mitral valve, or retrograde via the aortic valve. The retrograde approach tends to send the catheter towards the freewall, so it can be challenging to map the septum from this approach. The trans-septal approach provides easier access to the septum, but it can be difficult to reach the freewall from this approach.

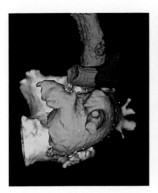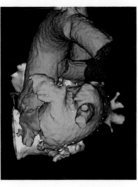

Figure 5.15 Mitral and tricuspid annuli. The mitral annulus is *not* lined up directly adjacent to the tricuspid annulus. The mitral sits more posteriorly; there is a portion of septum that separates the right *atrium* from the left *ventricle*.

Left meets right

Interestingly, the tricuspid and mitral annuli are not lined up with each other. If you think of the atria as up, and the ventricles as down, the MA is higher than the TA. This has an interesting implication: there is a place in the RA where you could poke a hole into the LVOT (not the LA) (Figure 5.15). Thus there is an RA/LA septum, an RA/LV septum, and an RV/LV septum.

Summary

- Atrial "coordinates": standard nomenclature applies easily to the ventricles but is confusing when applied to the atria. Anterior/superior vs. inferior/posterior, annular vs. posterior (actually "anti-annular"), septal vs. freewall. Beware: posterior can be used to refer to two different locations depending upon context.
- RA: RAA is anterior to the SVC–RA junction. Bachmann's bundle is anterior and septal to the SVC–RA junction. Lateral to the SVC–RA junction is the crista terminalis (endocardial)/sulcus terminalis (epicardial). The sinus node lies along the sulcus terminalis.
- The crista terminalis (CT) runs along the RA freewall and turns into the Eustachian ridge (ER) at the inferolateral aspect of the RA. The Eustachian ridge turns into the tendon of Todaro (TT) at the inferoseptal aspect of the RA (just above the CS os). The tendon of Todaro runs superiorly into the tricuspid annulus (TA).
- The cavo-tricuspid isthmus (CTI): the area between the TA and ER (typically narrowest isthmus in atrial flutter). The CTI can vary in width, can have thick trabeculae, and can be "pouch"-shaped.
- Triangle of Koch: bounded by TT, TA, and CS os (at floor). Contains the AV node (AVN), SP at the bottom, FP at the top; His arises from the top of the triangle and passes through the cartilaginous ring of the TA as the "penetrating bundle."
- The mitral annulus (MA) is offset from the tricuspid annulus such that there is an area of septum that separates RA from LV.
- Left atrium: there are four pulmonary veins; the superior veins are annular to the inferior veins, the roof slopes down from the left superior to the right superior PV. Veins can have separate or common ostia.
- There is an electrical junction between PV and LA; it is typically not circumferential.
- There is an anatomic junction between the LA and the PV antrum.
- The coronary sinus (CS) has its own musculature. CS musculature–atrial connections are to the RA at the CS os, to the LA along the LA floor. CS musculature ends at the Vieussens valve, where the CS turns into the great cardiac vein (GCV). Ventricular veins branching off the CS can make electrical connections to the LV, becoming posteroseptal epicardial pathways.

PART II

Doctor's-eye view (dealing with incomplete knowledge)

This book is divided into two parts, the first of which has described the heart and electrophysiology as if we "know all." We have been talking about our subject as if we know everything. We have described ion channel gates opening and closing, or cells exciting their neighbors, producing waves of propagation through the tissue in 3D. This all serves to build a foundation upon which we interpret the data we actually perceive when studying the heart. Thus, having built up the basic principles relevant to EP, we now turn to the second part of this book, which is told from the "doctor's-eye view." One of the greatest challenges to the practice of EP is translating the data that we observe – x-rays, electrograms, etc. – into a mental picture of activation waves propagating through the heart. It is only after we've made this translation that we can formulate hypotheses about what is happening, why, and what we can do about it.

In Part II we will discuss how to identify where you are in 3D space using tools like x-ray, ultrasound, electrograms, catheter movement, and 3D mapping systems. We'll discuss the relationship between the heart's electrical activity (the thing about which we care) and electrograms (the thing we get to see). We'll review some of the ideas of differential diagnostic pacing maneuvers; these largely involve combining our understanding of "how things work" with analytic reasoning to deduce information that we cannot directly acquire. The first part of this book was preparation; now the game truly begins.

The image-processing analogy for cardiac mapping

My colleague Jason Bates once proposed to me what he called "the image-processing analogy for cardiac mapping." It is a very helpful perspective from which to view mapping; it weaves an array of subjects into a very intuitive story about the challenges to creating interpretable maps.[1] The analogy goes like this:

Imagine that the electrical activity of the heart is an image that we want to take a picture of (or more aptly a video of). The spread of electrical activity across the 3D anatomy of the heart is the thing to be *imaged*, and the data we acquire does the *imaging*. Your map is the picture; your mapping "tools" are the camera. As in photography, if we use a very low-resolution camera we have a hard time making out what our picture *is*. We use large "mega-pixel" cameras because they make the picture much clearer. In the case of mapping, "pixels"

---

[1] I use the term "map" here in a very broad sense to include the formation of a mental map of cardiac electrical activity, using some measure of electrical activity and the anatomic locations from which this activity is recorded.

Understanding Clinical Cardiac Electrophysiology: A Conceptually Guided Approach, First Edition. Peter Spector.
© 2016 John Wiley & Sons, Inc. Published 2016 by John Wiley & Sons, Inc.
Companion website: www.wiley.com/go/spector/cardiac_electrophysiology

are analogous to electrodes/electrograms (the more the merrier). However, simply having a lot of pixels may not be sufficient. If your camera lens is out of focus, even a gazillion mega-pixel picture is uninterpretable. With poor focus the picture becomes "blurry"; colors from one pixel "bleed" into adjacent pixels. Focus is analogous to the spatial resolution of our electrodes. As we will see, electrograms and the heart's electrical activity are not one and the same. The excitation states of the cells that make up the heart are spatially discrete; a cell's currents are *at the location of that cell*. This is not what we measure clinically. These currents produce an electric potential field which spreads out through space; the potential field is *not confined to the location of the current that generated it*. We measure the potential field, not the heart's currents. Because the potential field is diffuse, it is basically a "blurred" view of the currents. Thus a "good" map requires an adequate number of pixels (number of electrodes) *and* adequate focus (spatial resolution of electrodes). Later we will discuss what "adequate" means in the context of mapping.

Before we discuss electrograms and the relation between electric currents and the electric field we begin with anatomy. How do we know where our pixels are?

6
Deducing anatomy

Using imaging to navigate the heart

The last chapter of Part I, *Anatomy for electrophysiologists*, was a quick listing of some anatomic points-of-interest from an EP perspective. But even if you have a complete mental image of the heart's 3D landscape, as an electrophysiologist you will never actually see it. You'll need to use several indirect data streams, each of which is inadequate, and combine these to decide "where you are." Our tools include fluoroscopy (with or without contrast), intracardiac ultrasound, 3D mapping technologies, pre-procedural imaging, and electrograms. Fluoroscopy (fluoro) is the anchor of the EP lab. Although much effort has been expended to allow low- (and sometimes no-) fluoro procedures, fluoro is the starting point for EP.

Fluoroscopy

The first thing you'll notice (I hope) when you look at fluoro is that you can't see the heart. There is a shadow of its margins but that's all. What you can see, quite prominently, is the catheters that you've placed in the heart. The first "trick" of anatomy-for-EP is making use of the catheters to identify cardiac anatomy. We frequently use the right and left anterior oblique projections (RAO and LAO) to "look" at the heart. These views are useful because they separate right from left (LAO) and atria from ventricles (RAO) (Figure 6.1). It is not uncommon to hear people say that LAO is 60° and RAO is −30°. This is not a very useful way to set up your fluoro cameras. These numbers reflect the camera's position relative to the *body*, but the heart can vary in its position relative to the body; it is much more useful to line up the cameras

with the *heart* (only then do you separate right and left, atria and ventricles).

So how *do* you set your camera angles?

RAO

The coronary sinus (CS) runs parallel to the mitral annulus (MA). If you place a catheter into the CS that catheter will run parallel to the MA. Thus if you line up the RAO camera such that the CS catheter is "foreshortened" you have set your angle relative to the heart. When set this way, "up" and to the left[1] are the atria, and "down" and to the right are the ventricles (Figure 6.1). How do you know the catheter is in the CS before you've set your camera angles? You simply set your angles by the body (roughly −30° and 60°) then cross from the IVC into the RV and "clock"[2] the catheter to bring it against the septum. Then pull back (towards the RA) while keeping gentle clockwise pressure. Until you cross the valve the septum will not allow the catheter to rotate leftward.[3] Once you reach the CS os, your catheter can enter the CS; you will see (and feel) the catheter turn leftward. At this point, advancing (with gentle clock) will bring you into the CS. You observe the movements of the catheter combined with the electrograms arising from its tip as your guide. At the beginning of this movement, when you're still far in the RV, you'll see ventricular

---

[1] As viewed on the fluoro screen.

[2] We will often use the short hand convention "clocking" and "counterclocking" for "placing clockwise (or counterclockwise) torque on a catheter."

[3] This actually introduces a very important concept in clinical EP. A final "data stream" at our disposal in the lab is the relationship between the forces we place on the catheter and the movement we observe with imaging. For example, when we try to clock the catheter yet see that the tip doesn't rotate we can deduce that something is physically precluding movement of the catheter tip.

Understanding Clinical Cardiac Electrophysiology: A Conceptually Guided Approach, First Edition. Peter Spector.
© 2016 John Wiley & Sons, Inc. Published 2016 by John Wiley & Sons, Inc.
Companion website: www.wiley.com/go/spector/cardiac_electrophysiology

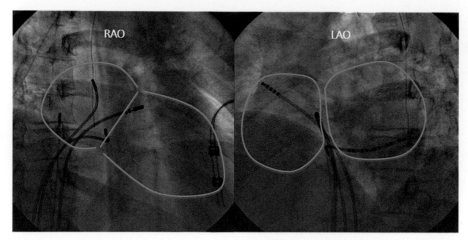

Figure 6.1 RAO and LAO projections. The RAO projection separates atria from ventricles. The LAO separates right from left.

electrograms (V) but no atrial electrograms (A). As you approach the tricuspid annulus (TA), you'll see A and V. At this point you are on the lookout for leftward catheter movement. While in the CS, you should see A and V "balance" (i.e., A and V of approximately equal amplitude).[4] If, once in the CS, you start to see only V on the distal CS electrodes, you have entered a ventricular branch; pulling back and redirecting will get you back to the CS.

LAO

In a fashion similar to the RAO, the LAO is set by lining a catheter up with the interventricular septum and then lining the LAO camera up so as to foreshorten that catheter. Again the trick is knowing how to line a catheter up with the septum (without directly seeing it). It turns out to be pretty easy. The triangle of Koch provides the answer. One side of the triangle is the tendon of Todaro (TT) and the other is the TA (Figure 6.2). Both are stiff structures not deformed by a catheter. If one places a catheter across the two, that catheter is lined up with the septum (i.e., separating right from left).

But how do you know you're lying across the TT/TA? The recorded electrograms tell you. When you record "the correct" His electrogram you know you are lying across the TT and TA. The important caveat here is the term "correct" electrogram; you have to be recording a His "below" (on the ventricular side of) the TT (Figure 6.3). It turns out one can record a prominent H

---

[4] Although in many patients the CS is so far towards the A that there is little or no V.

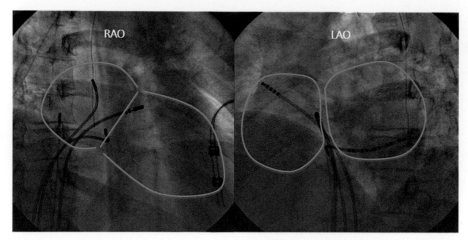

Figure 6.2 Setting the LAO camera angle. A CT image of the heart viewed from below. The coronary sinus (CS) is flanked by the tricuspid annulus (TA) and the tendon of Todaro (TT, red dots). A line connecting these two structures aligns with the septum. When the His catheter is placed across valve and held against the TT and TA (clockwise torque) it lines up with the septum. If we set the LAO angle such that it foreshortens the His catheter in this position, we have aligned LAO to the heart (instead of the body).

either above or below the TT. When above the tendon (meaning on the atrial side) your catheter sits in the annular-most portion of the fossa; the fossa is a distinctly deformable structure. So, with a catheter above the tendon, you can turn that catheter towards the left and it *is not lined up with the septum* (even though it records a large H) (Figure 6.3; see also Video 6.1).

When recording an H, how do you know if you're above or below the tendon? With the catheter below the tendon the proximal electrodes are in the triangle and

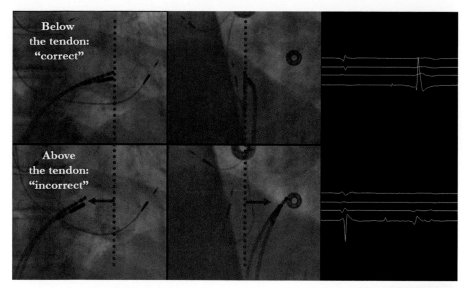

Figure 6.3 His catheter above and below the tendon of Todaro. (Top) With the His below the tendon (on the ventricular side) it aligns with the septum. Here it records A proximally and H and V distally. (Bottom) When the His catheter is above the tendon it can rotate leftwards; here it records large A distally.

the distal electrodes are in the ventricle. In this position the catheter records a small (or no) A proximally and a small H and large V distally (Figure 6.3). Above the tendon the catheter is very near the *left* ventricle (remember that the MA is above the TA); the catheter records a large A, large H, and large V. This is a seemingly very good place to put your His catheter; it gives you all the electrograms you want for differential diagnosis. There are, however, two downsides to placing the catheter above the tendon. First, it is not aligned with the septum and hence should *not* be used to set the LAO angle. Second, and more importantly, the catheter can slide over the fast pathway (which crosses over the TT superiorly) causing transient loss of FP conduction and rendering some arrhythmias transiently non-inducible.

Isocenter

X-ray is essentially a "shadow-gram".[5] It is easy to see that a catheter is pointed to the left or to the right of the screen; it is not possible to directly discern whether it is pointed towards or away from the camera. The RAO and LAO projections offer complementary information. Because the cameras are lined up 90° from one another, left and right in one view are towards and away in the other. As a result we often switch back and forth between

the RAO and LAO projections. When doing so it is very convenient to have the table (heart) at "isocenter." Isocenter is the table position at which the heart lies in the center of the x-ray beam *in both the RAO and LAO projections*. It is only very briefly amusing to watch a new fellow move the table every time they switch between RAO and LAO to re-center the heart.

Getting to isocenter is simple. With the camera in the RAO projection move the table side-to-side until the heart is in the center of the image. Now *don't* move it side-to-side any more. In the LAO raise or lower the table until the heart is centered (and don't move this again). This is isocenter … you are set for the rest of the case (Figure 6.4).

Trans-septal catheterization

While this book is not a recipe for how to do things and essentially leaves out any discussion of therapy or specific procedures, I am including a section on transseptal catheterization (TS) because it offers an excellent example of how we combine pieces of indirect information to find our "anatomic bearings." In the last 15–20 years it has become much easier (and hence routine) to use intracardiac ultrasound during TS. This has certainly reduced the incidence of complications. In this chapter we are not going to discuss ultrasound; if you understand

---

[5] Think hand-shadows making a rabbit.

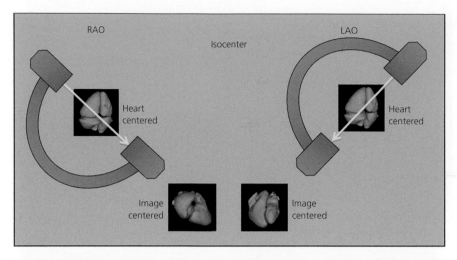

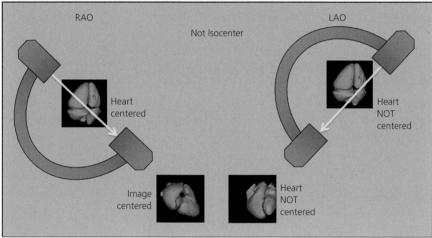

Figure 6.4 Isocenter. When the heart is in the middle of the x-ray beam in both RAO and LAO, the heart is at isocenter.

(and can perform) TS without ultrasound, you can certainly do it safely with ultrasound.

One fundamental principle of putting an 80 cm needle into a person's heart is "never move an uncovered needle forward, unless you're ready to make a hole." The term needle here must really be extended to include anything that can poke a hole through the heart or a blood vessel. This includes dilators and stiff sheaths. In fact even guide wires or catheters *when they are being advanced out of the end of a sheath* can perforate the heart, because they are being prevented, by the sheath, from bending over.[6] Most guide wires have a "j-curve" at their tip. As a result the "j" and not the tip is pushed against the

vessel/heart wall. However, when the wire first comes out of the dilator, it cannot bend into its "j"; under these circumstances, the tip *can* push against a wall (and perforate).

Crossing the fossa

The goal of trans-septal catheterization is to get a sheath to cross the septum so catheters can be placed in and out of the LA without "losing" access across the septum. To do this you have to make a hole (typically with a needle[7]). You then have to get a sheath across that hole. When your needle first crosses the septum, the hole is no wider than the needle. The sheath (which is much

---

[6] To avoid trouble it is wiser to get a catheter or wire to the tip of the sheath and then pull the sheath backward rather than advancing the catheter forward. Once the tip is "free" (to bend) it is much safer to push it forward.

[7] Sometimes the dilator alone can cross the septum. The septum can also be perforated using RF delivered to the tip of a wire on the fossa. The high current density at the tip of the very narrow wire creates a hole.

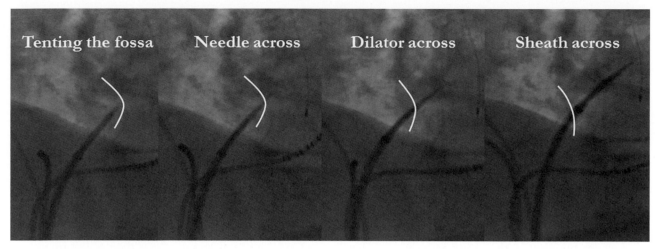

Tenting the fossa   Needle across   Dilator across   Sheath across

Figure 6.5 Crossing the fossa. (1) the needle "tents" the fossa; (2) the needle crosses, sheath and dilator remain on the right (the dilator and needle must be advanced together until the dilator has crossed the septum); (3) the needle and dilator are across; (4) the dilator has fully dilated the septum, the sheath is *ready* to cross.

wider) will not go through that hole. We therefore make the hole wider using a dilator. This is a stiff plastic straw that has a channel through its center (that the needle or wire can go through). The outer diameter of the dilator is small at the tip (not much wider than the needle) and gets progressively larger as you travel proximally down the first ~1.5 cm of its end. At this point the outer diameter of the dilator is equal to the inner diameter of the sheath. Once you have determined that the sheath/dilator/needle is in the fossa (see below) you advance the needle beyond the tip of the dilator (holding the sheath/dilator in place). If the needle doesn't cross the septum, then push the whole sheath/dilator/needle (as a unit) until the needle crosses.

How do you know when you've crossed the fossa? Basically you can usually feel it. Unless the needle just pushes straight across (relatively rare) you build pressure against the fossa. At first the fossa deviates leftward (away from your needle), causing "tenting" (Figure 6.5). Then there is typically a palpable "pop" as the needle makes a hole through the fossa (see Video 6.2). In addition to feeling this I (highly) recommend attaching a pressure transducer to the end of the needle that will allow measurement of the pressure through the tip (Figure 6.6).[8] This is a point where novices often make a frustrating

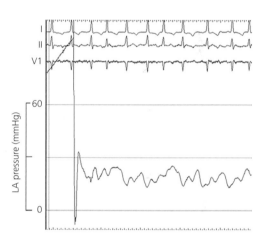

Figure 6.6 Pressure recorded through the tip of the TS needle. If you record pressure through the needle you can avoid dilating a hole in the wrong structure.

mistake. Having crossed the septum your needle is on the left but the dilator and sheath are still on the right. If you hold the needle fixed and push the dilator forward, the dilator will push the fossa wall back over the tip of the needle and you'll be back on the right (Figure 6.7; see also Video 6.3).

You must keep the relative positions of the needle and the dilator fixed while you get the tip of the dilator across the fossa.[9] This is a little dangerous, because the dilator meets resistance as it pushes against the fossa; when the dilator finally crosses it can "jump" leftward in

---

[8] You will feel a "pop" regardless of what wall you've just perforated. If the pressure is LA you've made the correct hole and can safely dilate that hole. If you see LV, aortic, or mediastinal pressure you can stop (i.e., not dilate) *before* you've turned a little hole into a really big hole.

---

[9] In other words, push the sheath/dilator/needle as a unit until the dilator has crossed the fossa.

the process. If this happens while the needle is sticking out of the end of the dilator, the needle can perforate the next wall it hits. It is important therefore (1) to check that the needle isn't pointing too posteriorly or too annularly (so there's maximum space after it jumps) and (2) to watch the pressure even after the needle enters the left atrium (if you see dampening you're against a wall (Figure 6.8); you don't want to push the needle in that direction). Once the *dilator* has crossed you can advance the dilator over the needle (by holding the needle fixed while advancing the dilator). When you feel less back-pressure (or when it appears that the dilator has moved pretty far leftward) you can hold the needle and dilator fixed while you advance the sheath into the LA. There is often a final "pop" as the sheath crosses. The last trick is to *not* pull the whole thing back into the RA when

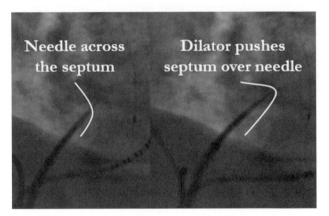

Figure 6.7 Advancing the dilator too soon. The needle must remain out of the end of the dilator until after the dilator has crossed the fossa, otherwise the dilator simply pushes the septum over the end of the needle (back on the right or into the middle of the septum).

removing the dilator and needle. You can watch the movement of the sheath as you begin to withdraw the dilator/needle, if it begins to bend (tip downward, "elbow" upward) it is probably not on the left. Stop, re-advance the dilator/needle, and then retry getting the sheath across.

Although we can't see the fossa we can see the sheath/dilator/needle. When we "push" the needle (from outside the body) we would like the upward force to be redirected leftward by the curve at the end of the needle (Figure 6.9). Sometimes, pushing causes the sheath/dilator/needle to move superiorly instead. Leftward movement from this superior position would result in entering the mediastinum above the LA. It is important to watch for leftward movement as we push the needle. If the needle moves superiorly, I remove it and place a bend about 15 cm proximal to the tip (Figure 6.10). This causes the "elbow" we've created to push against the IVC/RA junction and redirect the superior force from below into a leftward force at the tip.

It may seem that none of this has much to do with using indirect information to determine anatomic information. In fact we've already talked about some classic indirect information. When you make use of how the catheter feels or what the sheath looks like on fluoro you are using indirect information. We can't see the fossa; we infer its condition by interpreting feedback like bending of the sheath/dilator/needle or the look and feel of a "pop." The pressure measurement from the tip is also indirect information about the anatomic location of the needle tip.

In the preceding description I skipped over something important – how to get the needle into the fossa

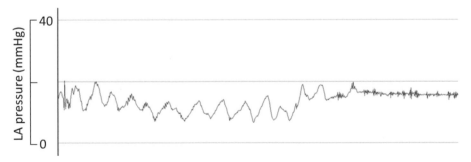

Figure 6.8 Pressure dampens when the needle contacts a surface. If the pressure tracing dampens as you attempt to push the sheath across the septum, it means that your tip is touching some structure. If there is a jump as the sheath crosses it could cause the needle to perforate through a far wall of the LA. Therefore if you see dampening while doing your trans-septal, readjust the needle angle to relieve the pressure.

Needle moves left   Needle moves up   Needle moves left

Shaft pushes
against IVC RA
junction

Figure 6.9 Ensuring that the needle moves leftward. Sometimes advancing the needle into the body causes it to rise up over the limbus rather than moving leftward across the septum. Placing a slight bend in the shaft of the needle ~10–15 cm from the tip can result in this angle deflecting off the IVC–RA junction and pushing the needle tip leftward.

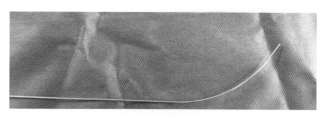

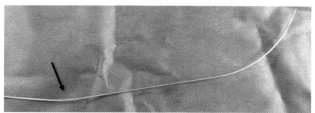

Figure 6.10 IVC curve. Placing a small bend in the proximal portion of the needle can help to force it leftward when advanced into the body (instead of traveling upward).

(and know that you're there). Here we use a great deal of indirect information.

Getting to the fossa

As we discussed above, you never want to move anything that might make a hole forward until you are in the fossa; so how do you get from the groin to the fossa without moving "pokey" stuff forward? We start by placing a wire through the sheath and dilator and advancing into the SVC over the wire. The curved wire tip prevents the dilator from pushing against a wall. Once in the SVC we remove the wire and place the needle *inside* the dilator, proximal to its tip (and flush it). Next we orient our sheath/dilator/needle so that when we pull it down, it will fall into the fossa. To do so we aim

it leftward and slightly annular. Having set the camera angles this means leftward in the LAO and midway between completely foreshortened and rightward (annular) in the RAO (Figure 6.11).

If you line up too annularly before you pull, the sheath/dilator/needle will end up in the triangle of Koch, and it will be difficult to clock it across the TT into the fossa. In addition, clocking across the TT places a great deal of pressure on the fast pathway. If you line up/pull too posteriorly, it is relatively smooth to counterclock into the fossa. If you watch in the LAO as you pull down, you will see that while in the SVC the sheath/dilator/needle-tip extends relatively far leftward until it's been pulled into the RA. As the sheath/dilator/needle-tip crosses over the limbus (which is too firm to be moved by the needle) it is deflected rightward. As you pull further, you drop over the limbus into the fossa; the tip jumps leftward again (see Chapter 5, Figure 5.6).

If you see the sheath/dilator/needle foreshorten as you pull, this could mean either that it has turned too far posteriorly or too far annularly. It is much more common to turn in the annular direction. Thus if you see foreshortening you can add a little more clockwise torque, "on the fly," without stopping and stepping on RAO.

Once you drop below the limbus you need to confirm that you are in the fossa before you push the needle. Pushing from too posterior places you in the mediastinum; too annular, in the LVOT; annular/superior – the aorta; annular/inferior – the CS; too high – above the LA; and too low – below the LA. I recommend "just right."

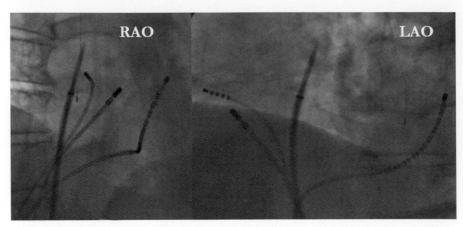

Figure 6.11 Needle position in the SVC. When preparing to pull the needle from the IVC into the fossa, it should be between pointing toward the ventricle and completely foreshortened in the RAO, and pointing leftward (right side of image) in the LAO.

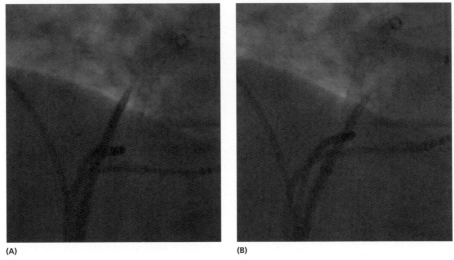

(A)   (B)

Figure 6.12 Finding the middle of the fossa. Clockwise torque on the trans-septal "opens it up," the tip moves farther to the left: note that in panel (A) the tip is to the right of the other sheath, in panel (B) it is to the left. With further rotation the trans-septal began to foreshorten again (the point at which it is most "open" indicates the center of the fossa).

How can you tell where to push? The fossa is thin (hence typically easy to cross) and as such it will "tent" when the stiff sheath/dilator/needle pushes against it. This is partially why the sheath/dilator/needle is able to move leftward. Imagine you have a tent that is fixed to the ground all around the edges of the floor. If you place a pole in the middle you can push it upwards maximally. As you move the pole towards either side of the tent it cannot stick up quite as high. If you were looking horizontally (parallel to the ground) you would see the pole maximally "opened" when it is in the center of the tent and see it foreshorten when it is moved toward either side. Thus, watch how "open" the sheath/dilator/needle is in the LAO as you clock (or counterclock). If you are at the middle of the fossa, movement in either direction will cause the sheath/dilator/needle to foreshorten. If you see the sheath/dilator/needle "open" with clock, you *were* too annular (etc.) (Figure 6.12; see also Video 6.4).

Summary

- Have a 3D map of cardiac anatomy in your head.
- Use electrograms, fluoroscopy, ultrasound, and mapping to register your mental map with the data you can see.

- Fluoroscopy:
  - RAO allows you to distinguish atria from ventricles.
  - LAO allows you to distinguish left from right.
- To set the RAO angle: foreshorten the CS catheter.
- To set the LAO angle: foreshorten the His catheter, with the His below the tendon of Todaro (small A, His and large V distally).
- Isocenter: table position where the heart is in the center of both the LAO and the RAO beams.
- Finding isocenter: set RAO by moving the table side to side; set LAO by moving the table up and down.

7

Electrical activity, electrodes, and electrograms

The thing with which electrophysiologists concern themselves is the spread of excitation through the heart. This means the distribution of current through the tissue over time. One of the biggest hurdles to the practice of EP is that we do not (and cannot) directly see propagation through the heart. Instead we look at the magnitude of the electric potential field at our intracardiac electrodes (i.e., **electrograms**) and extrapolate from this how propagation spreads through the heart. If we are to understand EP via electrograms it is incumbent upon us to understand the relationship between (1) the heart's electrical activity, (2) the potential field it generates, and (3) the electrodes we use to measure the potential field. We don't quite record propagation with electrograms, we deduce it.

Let's begin with a ridiculously simple scenario: a single charged particle surrounded by empty space. A charged particle produces a potential field in a similar way that a mass produces a gravitational field. In fact, you can think of electrogram interpretation somewhat like trying to understand the distribution of *mass* when the only measuring device you have access to is a scale (i.e., measurements of the magnitude of the gravitational field). In each case (gravity and potential field) the magnitude of the field decreases with distance from the source as $1/r$. We will delve into the mathematical nature of this relationship in a moment, but at the outset let me state: armed with a complete measurement of the potential field (at *all* points in space) and knowledge of the mathematical relationship between electric current and the electric potential field, we could calculate the heart's electrical activity (the current source distribution) *perfectly*. The challenge, the source of ambiguity, is that we do not have infinite measurements of the potential field. We have perhaps 80, somewhat inadequate,

measurements; we are limited by the number of electrodes and by the geometry of those electrodes.

As described in the introduction to Part II, electrograms are like a blurred version of local current. In a blurred picture the colors at any given location "bleed" into neighboring locations. This is directly analogous to the spreading through space of the potential field around a current source. The location of the heart's currents is sharply demarcated; current exists where cells are excited and doesn't spread beyond these excited cells.[1] The potential field, on the other hand, extends (infinitely) outward from the current source.

Cardiac excitation isn't as simple as a single current source. At any moment in time currents are distributed throughout the heart. The current at *each* location contributes to the potential field. How exactly does each of these currents contribute to an electrogram? Luckily, we can consider the impact of each site independently and simply add them all together (a principle called superposition). The larger the current, and the closer that current is to a recording site, the larger its contribution to the electrogram. Consider the distribution of currents as a wave of excitation propagates through the heart. At the leading edge of excitation (where cells that have just been depolarized are immediately adjacent to cells that are at rest) there is a very large voltage gradient over a very short distance. This means that the local current density is (by far) highest at the leading edge of excitation; current is flowing all along the wave but the local voltage gradients (and hence current densities) behind the leading edge are much

---

[1] Don't mistake *propagation* (the sequential excitation of myocytes) for current being spatially unconstrained. At any moment current exists in discrete locations.

Understanding Clinical Cardiac Electrophysiology: A Conceptually Guided Approach, First Edition. Peter Spector.
© 2016 John Wiley & Sons, Inc. Published 2016 by John Wiley & Sons, Inc.
Companion website: www.wiley.com/go/spector/cardiac_electrophysiology

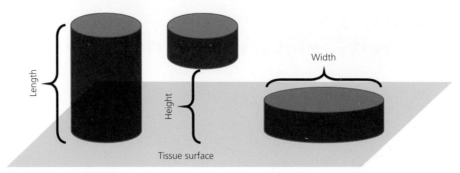

Figure 7.1 Electrode geometry and spatial resolution. As electrode length increases, resolution decreases (average height increases). As height increases the difference in distance between cells immediately beneath and those to the side of the electrode diminishes. As electrode width increases, footprint increases (i.e., there are a greater number of cells that are directly beneath the electrode).

smaller. It is a reasonable simplification to think of the current source as if it were just the leading edge traveling through space. The leading edge is essentially a positive charge (excited cell) adjacent to a negative charge (unexcited cell); a positive charge adjacent to a negative charge is called a dipole. Mathematically, if we make calculations based upon a moving dipole the problem of calculating potential fields becomes much simpler yet retains a very close relationship to the actual size of the potential field.

The potential deceases with the distance from a single charge (remember $1/r$, above); how does it decrease with distance from a **dipole**? It diminishes (essentially) with the *square* of the distance ($1/r^2$). The result is that the electrogram amplitude decreases pretty quickly as the distance between the wave and the electrode increases. There is one final point. I've been playing fast and loose with the terms "charge" and "current"; in the preceding paragraph I've used them as if they were interchangeable. The mathematical derivation is long and unnecessary for understanding what we need to know for electrogram interpretation, but it turns out that, effectively, you *can* swap charge and current in the electrogram story.

Intracardiac recording and spatial resolution

If the electric potential was measurable at the source current and was *zero* everywhere else, spatial resolution would be perfect (i.e., electrodes would record only local activity). At the other extreme, if potential didn't diminish *at all* with distance, spatial resolution would be absent (there would be no means to discern the location of a current source *based upon electrogram amplitude*).

But, as it turns out, potential does diminish with distance. This means that there is some blurring: an electrode records activity from the tissue immediately beneath it *and from the region nearby*. **Spatial resolution** is a measure of the size of the "nearby region" that contributes to an electrogram.

Electrode spatial resolution is dependent upon several things. You can already deduce one of these: **height** above the tissue. Think about the EKG, which shows electrical activity from all parts of the heart (roughly) equally, while intracardiac electrodes preferentially show "local" activity. This is not because the electrodes are different, rather it's because the geometric relationship between the location of the electrodes and the location of the electrical activity is different. When an electrode is high above the heart (e.g., EKG) it is roughly the same *distance* from all portions of the heart – whereas an electrode on the heart's surface is much closer to some cells than it is to other cells.

The **size** of the electrode impacts resolution as well. A *wider*[2] electrode has a larger "footprint" (i.e., there is a greater area of tissue that is "local": Figure 7.1). But why does the *length*[3] of the electrode impact its resolution? This may seem a little less obvious at first glance. To explain the impact of length we must note that an electrode is a conductor and that *there cannot be a potential gradient on the surface of a conductor*.[4] The result is that the potential measured by an electrode is equal to the average of the potentials that would be

---

[2] Its extent parallel to the plane of the tissue.
[3] Its extent perpendicular to the plane of the tissue.
[4] If there were a voltage gradient, current would flow until the gradient was absent (i.e., the potential is equal everywhere on a conductor).

recorded at each location on that electrode. Because the potential on the entire electrode is the same there is zero spatial resolution *within* the electrode.[5] So, why does electrode length matter? The taller an electrode is, the greater the average height of that electrode above the tissue. Because spatial resolution decreases with height, as average height increases resolution decreases.

Recording configuration and spatial resolution

By "recording configuration" I mean bipolar vs. unipolar. In reality there is no such thing as a unipolar potential measurement. Any recording is the difference in potential between two electrodes. "Unipolar" refers to a bipolar recording in which one of the two electrodes (the "indifferent" electrode) is far enough from the heart that it essentially records zero potential. Under these circumstances a "unipolar" electrogram effectively displays only the potential of the electrode in the heart (the "index" electrogram minus zero "equals" the index electrogram). When we say "bipolar," we are referring to a recording in which both electrodes are close enough to the tissue to be measuring a non-zero potential. In this case the bipolar electrogram is truly the difference between the unipolar electrograms that would be recorded at each of the electrode sites (Figure 7.2). If the electrodes "see" the exact same thing there is no difference and the electrogram is zero (a flat line). This impacts the spatial resolution because as a source moves farther away from a pair of electrodes it looks ever more similar to both electrodes. Therefore when you subtract one from the other the difference decreases, i.e., far-field signals are small (Figure 7.2).

As two electrodes are moved closer together (decreased inter-electrode spacing) the "far-field" signals look more and more the same to each of them. Therefore **inter-electrode spacing** is inversely proportional to the spatial resolution of bipolar electrodes.

This capacity to diminish far-field signal enhances the effective spatial resolution of bipolar electrodes. There is a "catch": bipolar electrodes have a larger "footprint" than unipolar electrodes (Figure 7.3) and their amplitude is

---

[5] By "within" here I mean anywhere along its surface; the potential is actually zero *inside* a conductor.

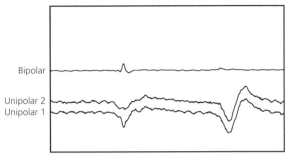

Figure 7.2 Bipolar vs. unipolar spatial resolution. A bipolar signal is generated by subtracting the unipolar signal of one electrode from the unipolar signal of the other. Therefore things that "look the same" to both electrodes (i.e., things far away) are subtracted away, while things that look different (i.e., things close by) remain. Note that the first deflection is seen on the unipolar and the bipolar electrograms (because there is a difference between the two unipolar signals). The second deflection is present only on the unipolar signals (there is essentially nothing on the bipolar tracing) because the signal is the same on both unipolar tracings. Also note in this figure that there is much more "noise" on the unipolar tracings than the bipolar tracings (the noise is the same on both unipolars).

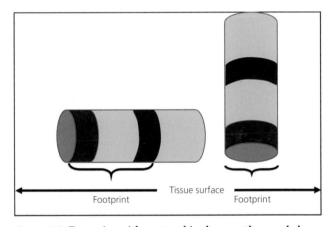

Figure 7.3 Footprint with contact bipole vs. orthogonal close unipole. The net surface area of electrode in contact with the tissue varies depending upon catheter orientation.

"direction-dependent." The footprint effect is pretty straightforward, but what does direction-dependence mean? The geometric relationship between the electrodes and a wave front of excitation (the source) is such that when a wave approaches along the direction of the axis between the electrodes (Figure 7.4) the distance between the source and each electrode is maximally different and the potential is largest. Compare this with a wave approaching perpendicular to the long axis between the electrodes. In this case the source is at all times equidistant from both electrodes, hence the difference is

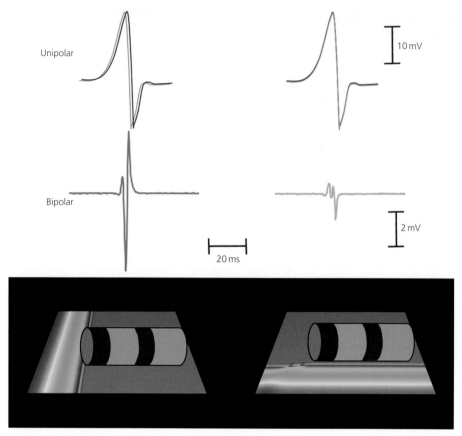

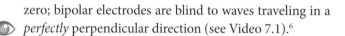

Figure 7.4 Direction-dependence of the bipolar electrogram. When a wave front approaches the electrodes in long axis the difference between the electrodes is maximal and hence the signal amplitude is largest. When the wave front approaches perpendicular to the electrodes it looks the same to both and the signal is smallest (with complete symmetry, the electrogram is zero).

zero; bipolar electrodes are blind to waves traveling in a *perfectly* perpendicular direction (see Video 7.1).[6]

Orthogonal close unipolar

If you take a bipolar electrode pair and orient it "normal" to the plane of the tissue (Figure 7.5C) its electrogram properties are markedly altered. It becomes *direction-independent* and its spatial resolution is improved (compared with a contact bipolar). We call this orientation "orthogonal close unipolar" (OCU) because it is *orthogonal* to the tissue, only *one electrode* is in contact with the tissue (unipolar), and the indifferent electrode is very *close* (as opposed to being in the IVC, for example). The impact of this geometric orientation is

(1) reduced footprint,[7] (2) near-field/far-field discrimination,[8] and (3) direction independence.[9]

Quantifying spatial resolution

The qualitative notion of spatial resolution is fairly easily understood: it is the size of the region that an electrode "sees." In order to compare different electrodes and recording configurations it is useful to have a quantitative measure of spatial resolution. How can we quantify spatial resolution? If you think of an electrode's spatial resolution as the area of tissue that falls within the recording region of that electrode, then you might imagine that resolution could be quantified as the size of that region. One challenge with that approach is that the

---

[6] In practice wave fronts aren't perfectly perpendicular to electrode pairs, and hence electrogram amplitude (and morphology) depend upon wave/electrode orientation, but deflections aren't completely absent when the wave front is "perpendicular."

[7] Only one electrode rather than two.
[8] Like any bipolar electrode pair.
[9] The electrodes have the same geometric relationship to waves coming from any direction.

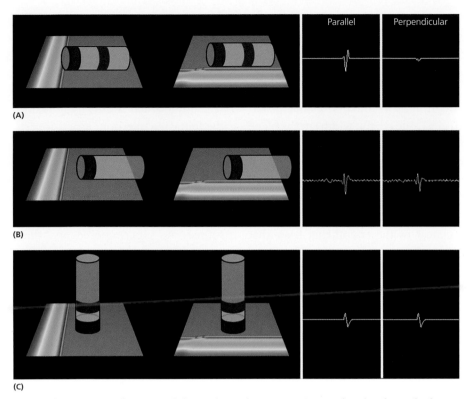

Figure 7.5 Impact of wave direction as a function of electrode configuration. Contact bipolar electrodes have improved spatial resolution over unipolar recordings but are impacted by wave direction. Orthogonal unipolar electrograms have the improved resolution of bipolar signals (plus a smaller footprint) without the direction-dependence.

recording region is not sharply circumscribed; there isn't a point at which the tissue changes from contributing-to-an-electrogram to not-contributing. If you were to think of the recording region like a circle of light created by a flashlight, that circle would be infinite in radius but the intensity of light would fall off with distance from the light's center. So how *do* we define and quantify the resolution of an electrode? One approach would be to arbitrarily define the size of the recording region as the radial distance at which the electrogram amplitude is 50% of its maximum. Then we just measure the distance to *that* location. The morphology of an electrogram is dependent, in part, on the electrode recording configuration. Let's discuss each configuration separately.

Examination of a unipolar electrogram reveals a signal that grows as a source gets closer to the electrode, reaches a peak, then rapidly transitions to a maximally negative deflection, and finally, as the source recedes, returns to baseline. One can measure the radial distance at which the amplitude of the electrogram decreases to 50% of its maximum (Figure 7.6A).[10] The morphology

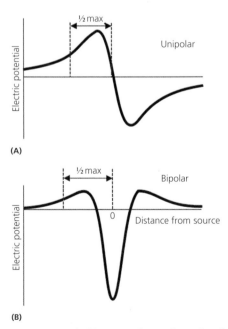

Figure 7.6 Distance to half-maximal signal amplitude. The distance from the center of the electrode to the location where the signal amplitude has decreased by 50% of its maximum value.

---

[10] After first increasing to its peak.

of a bipolar electrogram has two peaks and a trough (Figure 7.6B) (the trough actually has the largest absolute amplitude). For the purposes of this discussion we will measure the distance to half-maximal amplitude *of the positive peaks*.

Applying these definitions we find that spatial resolution decreases with electrode height, width (in the plane of the tissue), length (perpendicular to the plane of the tissue), and, for bipolar recordings, inter-electrode spacing (Figure 7.7). Height has the largest impact of all the electrode characteristics influencing resolution. Unless one uses plunge electrodes, electrode height is limited by the thickness of the endothelial layer that separates the heart's surface from myocytes. Thus even

an infinitely small electrode is limited by the resolution constraints of height.

The pragmatic goal of improved spatial resolution is better discrimination between near-field and far-field signals. There is another way that we can quantify resolution which is directly linked to this goal. We ask the following question: if two sources start at the same location (i.e., are superimposed) and are incrementally moved apart, how far apart can they be before you are able to discern that there are two separate sources (rather than one)? This can be calculated using the correlation between the electrogram recorded when the sources are superimposed and that recorded as they are moved apart (Figure 7.8). At first there is a perfect

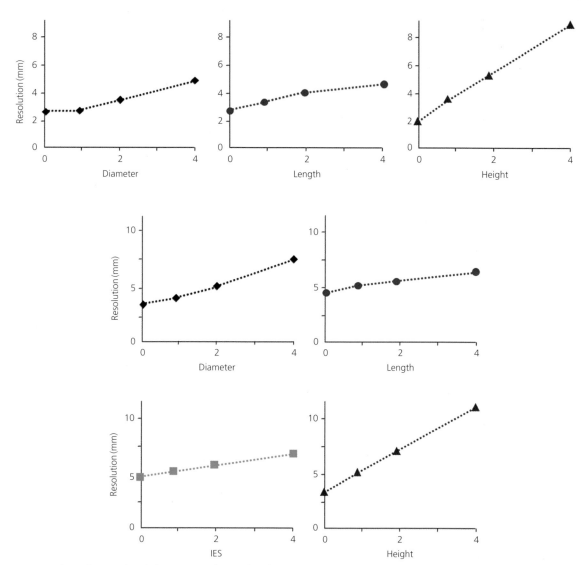

Figure 7.7 Spatial resolution. (Top) the impact of unipolar electrode diameter, length, and height on spatial resolution. (Bottom) the impact of bipolar electrode diameter, length, inter-electrode spacing (IES), and height on spatial resolution.

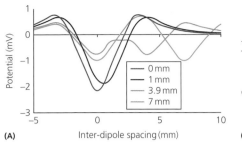

(A)   Inter-dipole spacing (mm)

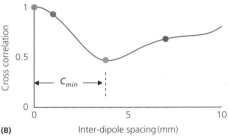

(B)   Inter-dipole spacing (mm)

Figure 7.8 **Discerning two sources as a function of inter-source separation.** (A) Calculated bipolar electrograms generated by two dipoles separated by 0, 1, 3.9, and 7 mm. (B) cross-correlation between single-dipole and double-dipole electrograms as a function of inter-dipole distance (colors correspond to spacing in (A)). The minimum cross-correlation (i.e., maximum ability to distinguish) is shown (C_{min}).

correlation, 1.0 (no ability to discriminate at all), and correlation decreases as the sources are separated. One can then simply measure the distance at which correlation decreases to 0.5.[11]

There is yet another, very pragmatic, way to quantify the ability to distinguish near-field from far-field signals. One can separate near and far sources in *time* (so there is no overlap of electrograms) and then measure the amplitude of the far-field signal. When we do this for the unipolar, orthogonal close unipolar, and contact bipolar recording configurations, the greatest resolution is seen with the OCU (Figure 7.9).

Calculating electrical activity from electrograms

There is a specific mathematical relationship between current and its potential field … So why can't we just mathematically derive the tissue currents from our electrogram measurements? The answer is a little nuanced but in fact is fairly straightforward. The process of deriving the currents from the electrograms is called deconvolution (don't worry about the exact meaning of that word). The relationship between current distribution and *an* electrogram measurement is "non-

Figure 7.9 **Far field signal as a function of electrode configuration.** The first deflection is A, the second is far-field V. Compare the relative amplitude of the first and second deflections with the different configurations; the bipolar and orthogonal close unipolar (OCU) signals have a much smaller far-field signal (relative to the first near-field deflection).

unique." This means that there are multiple different sizes/locations of currents that could result in the *same* electrogram. Imagine, by way of analogy, that we were trying to deduce the size and location of a mass from the amplitude of the gravitational field measured at a given location. One would be unable to determine whether there was a cannon ball 5 feet away or a planet 5 million miles away (or any of an *infinite* number of other combinations of size and distance). What if we made a second measurement of the gravitational field in a different location? For example, what if we moved

---

[11] Interestingly, if one continues to separate the sources beyond a point of minimum correlation, the correlation actually begins to improve again (Figure 7.8). This is because the electrogram from two superimposed sources is identical to that of a single source, and as the sources are separated there is a fusion between the electrograms of two sources with diminishing overlap. Once the sources are separated enough that the first and second "electrograms" no longer overlap, the first electrogram correlates very well with the superimposed electrogram (Figure 7.8).

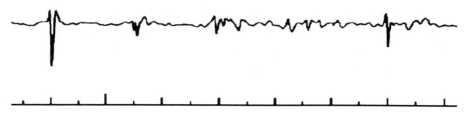

Figure 7.10 Complex fractionated atrial electrograms. Note that, due to varying spatiotemporal frequency, electrograms are organized (first complex) and then fractionated (middle of tracing).

our scale 10 feet in the direction from which gravity is pulling on our scale? We could certainly distinguish between the cannon ball (at 5 feet) and the planet. If it was the cannon ball all along then we would measure the same pull but in the opposite direction from our first measurement site; if it was a planet all along then the direction of pull would remain the same and the amplitude would increase a little. You can imagine that the uncertainty of our deduction increases as the number and distribution of currents increases. When we record electrograms there are lots of currents distributed over a very complex 3D landscape. If we were to make an infinite number of measurements of the potential field (at all points in space) we could identify exactly what the current size and distribution was. But, the fewer electrograms we record the greater the uncertainty of our calculation. The utility of deconvolution is a function of the number of measurements made. In order for deconvolution of electrograms to offer improvement over plain old electrograms we need a lot of electrodes. The number required depends upon the spatial complexity of the heart's electrical activity. For the most part you will not encounter deconvolution in clinical practice. But it is worthwhile to at least know about its existence.

Spatial resolution and electrogram fractionation

A lot has been made of "complex fractionated atrial electrograms" (CFAE) (Figure 7.10) in the last decade or so. There are many who use "CFAE" as a guide to ablation of atrial fibrillation. Obviously the logic in using electrogram morphology for choosing ablation targets is that this morphology identifies a site crucial to the initiation or maintenance of AF. Before assigning a specific significance to fractionation it is useful to understand exactly what fractionation *is* and how it's generated.

Basically fractionation is multiple nearly-superimposed deflections.[12] So, fractionation is caused by anything that results in multiple nearly-superimposed deflections.[13] When tissue (a group of cells) is depolarized in a single organized wave there is a steady variation in the electrogram deflection. Other than the triphasic morphology of a bipolar signal there are not multiple peaks and valleys (Figure 7.10: first complex). When there are uncoordinated activations of the cells in the recording region of an electrode, that electrode's electrogram will register multiple deflections. These deflections can range from completely superimposed (no offset of activation timing) through fractionated (partially offset) to completely separate (completely offset). So, fractionation requires dissociation of electrical activation of cells *within the recording region of an electrode*, and partially offset timing of these activations.

Tissue activation patterns and electrograms

Consider a few examples of dissociated cells and the electrograms they produce. First imagine laterally dissociated cells (basically parallel columns of cells that are not electrically connected) which are activated in parallel (Figure 7.11A; see also Video 7.2). Here we have dissociation but no temporal offset, and as a result no fractionation. If we create serial activation of these same parallel cell groups, the activation of the groups *is* temporally offset and multiple deflections result (Figure 7.11B; see also Video 7.2). In general terms *any- thing* that causes spatiotemporal variation of activation within the recording region of an electrode(s) will result in fractionation. Examples include patchy scar and

---

[12] If the deflections were entirely superimposed there would be only a single deflection and hence no fractionation.
[13] duh.

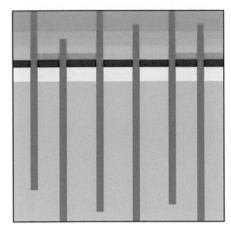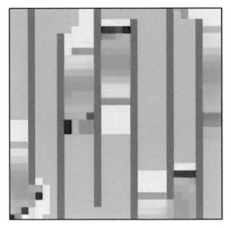

Figure 7.11 **Spatiotemporal variability.** Spatial variability occurs when cells are electrically separated (in space) but activated at the same time (in parallel). Spatiotemporal variability occurs when cells are separated in space and in time.

interstitial fibrosis (i.e., structural dissociation of groups of cells) and the boundary between waves in multi-wavelet reentry (i.e., functional dissociation of groups of cells).

It is important to note that this dissociation only results in electrogram fractionation if it occurs *within the recording region of the electrode(s)*. Because the recording region of an electrode varies with its configuration (i.e., its spatial resolution), fractionation must vary with spatial resolution as well (see Video 7.3).

If spatiotemporal variation *and* temporal variation alone can both cause fractionation, how can we distinguish which type of tissue activation underlies a fractionated electrogram? One way to distinguish spatiotemporal variation from temporal variation is to look for spatial resolution-dependence. Temporal variation alone will generate repetitive deflections regardless of whether one records from 1,000,000 cells or 1 cell, i.e., the fractionation due to temporal variation is *independent of spatial resolution*. Spatiotemporal variation on the other hand is spatial-resolution-dependent, and therefore the demonstration that a fractionated electrogram is spatial-resolution-dependent defines that fractionation as resulting from spatiotemporal variation.

Summary

- Electrical currents in the heart and electrograms are not the same thing.
- Currents create an electric potential field that surrounds the heart; this is what electrograms measure.
- Electrograms are effectively a blurred version of cardiac currents.
- Electric potential decreases with distance from a current source; electrograms decrease in amplitude with distance from the heart.
- The potential field at any point in space (e.g., at an electrode) is a simple summation of that which would be generated (individually) by all the currents in the heart – a principle called superposition.
- Propagation waves can be approximated as moving dipoles. We largely "see" only the wave *front*, not the wave tail; hence electrograms reflect activation, not recovery.
- Spatial resolution: the size of the tissue area that effectively contributes to an electrogram.
- Spatial resolution is proportional to an electrode's size, height above the tissue, configuration (unipolar vs. bipolar), and (for bipolar) inter-electrode spacing.
- The orthogonal close unipolar configuration (a bipolar electrode pair oriented perpendicular to the plane of the tissue surface) has the best spatial resolution and its amplitude is direction-independent.
- Electrogram fractionation results when the cells within an electrode's recording region are not acting in unison. Fractionation is a function of the ratio of tissue spatiotemporal variation and electrode spatial resolution.

8

Electrogram analysis: understanding electrogram morphology

Electrograms are the window into EP; they are the lens through which we see the heart's electrical activity. As we've been discussing, the thing we want to know about is the spread of activation through the heart, but this is not the thing we measure. In order to accurately interpret electrograms we must understand the relationships between currents in the heart, the potential field that they generate, and the impact of electrode size, shape, and configuration on electrograms. The details of those relationships were discussed in Chapter 7; here we will concern ourselves with the consequences.

Electrograms vs. EKGs

Electrograms measure changes in the potential field as seen from a given electrode or electrodes. These changes are dominated by the leading edge of activation. Thus when you look at electrograms you are largely looking at excitation/depolarization (as opposed to recovery/repolarization), specifically "local" activation. Before we dive into intracardiac electrograms let's take a moment to discuss the surface EKG. The EKG measures gradients in potential across the heart. For example we see a QRS while the ventricles are depolarizing (i.e., while some but not all ventricular myocytes are excited) but the EKG returns to baseline once all cells have been excited (we see a flat ST segment). We only see a new deflection (the T wave) when some areas of the ventricle have repolarized but others have not. Also note that the surface electrodes are far from the heart, so there must be a fairly large amount of current in order to generate a visible deflection on the EKG. We don't see sinus node depolarization (the sinus node tissue is too small

and depolarizes too slowly to generate a visible signal). The P wave begins when activation has left the sinus node and has excited a sufficiently large number of atrial myocytes. Similarly, as propagation traverses the His–Purkinje system (HPS) we see no deflection on the EKG. The QRS begins *after* activation has exited the HPS at the Purkinje–myocyte junctions *and* depolarized a sufficiently large group of ventricular myocytes to generate a detectable deflection on the body surface. You can actually detect the discrepancy between the time-of-first-myocyte-depolarization and the first-deflection-of-the-QRS when mapping accessory pathways during pre-excitation. Earliest ventricular activity, seen from inside the heart, precedes the onset of the delta wave. In fact this discrepancy is larger with right-sided pathways which insert into the thinner right ventricle and hence have to spread farther before they've "recruited" enough mass of myocardium to cause an EKG deflection.[1]

It's worth taking a moment to examine the relationship between the QRS-T complex and the cellular action potential. The QRS is larger and sharper than the T wave because the potential gradient is larger and occurs more abruptly during depolarization than during repolarization (Figure 8.1). Similarly, with intracardiac recordings the activation wave causes a larger sharper deflection than does the repolarization wave. In fact the repolarization wave causes a deflection so small that it is lost in the baseline "noise." This is particularly true in the atrium,

---

[1] You can think of the thinner RV as being two-dimensional, so as propagation spreads the number of excited cells grows with *area* (i.e., as πr^2). In the thicker LV the number of cells increases in three dimensions, as a *volume* (i.e., as $4/3\pi r^3$).

Understanding Clinical Cardiac Electrophysiology: A Conceptually Guided Approach, First Edition. Peter Spector.
© 2016 John Wiley & Sons, Inc. Published 2016 by John Wiley & Sons, Inc.
Companion website: www.wiley.com/go/spector/cardiac_electrophysiology

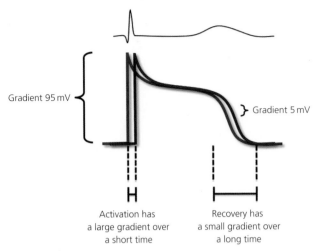

Gradient 95 mV

Gradient 5 mV

Activation has
a large gradient over
a short time

Recovery has
a small gradient over
a long time

Figure 8.1 Recording depolarization and repolarization on the EKG. The ventricular depolarization wave generates a larger signal (QRS) than the repolarization wave (T wave) due to a larger potential gradient over a shorter time. Atrial action potentials are shaped more like a triangle (ventricular action potentials are somewhat square) and hence there is no discernible "atrial T wave." (Blue and red action potentials represent the earliest and latest ventricular cells excited.)

because the atrial action potentials are shaped like a triangle while ventricular action potentials are shaped more like a square (Figure 8.2).[2]

Electrograms

In subsequent chapters we'll be discussing interpretation of *groups of electrograms*, i.e., electrograms recorded from multiple electrodes on multiple catheters. We will consider how to glean information by comparing electrograms with each other (e.g., activation sequence). In this chapter we'll be talking about analysis of individual electrograms and what information we can discern from them. Typically we record unipolar and bipolar electrograms in the EP lab; these provide complementary information, and we'll discuss both.

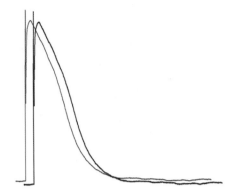

Figure 8.2 Atrial action potentials. Atrial action potentials are very triangular in shape, and hence the repolarization gradient is small and prolonged.

Unipolar electrograms

Imagine an electrode sitting on quiescent tissue with a wave of activation propagating towards it from a distance. At first the distance between the wave and the electrode is large enough that we record no potential. Remember we are measuring the difference between the potential recorded at the reference (remote) and the index electrode; at this point both see roughly the same thing (nothing) and the difference is zero (baseline). As the wave gets closer the potential field at the index electrode begins to grow and the electrogram slowly deviates upward from baseline. The electrogram grows with an increasingly steep slope as the wave gets closer.[3] As the wave front passes the electrode the amplitude of the electrogram diminishes, now with ever-decreasing slope. Also, because the leading edge is like a dipole, as it approaches, the electrode "sees" the positive current (upward deflection) and while it recedes the electrode sees the negative current (downward deflection).[4] Thus a unipolar electrogram records an upward deflection that increases its slope progressively to a peak, a rapid transition to a maximally negative deflection, and then the amplitude diminishes (with an ever-decreasing slope) (Figure 8.3).

---

[2] There is a technique (activation recovery interval, ARI) for grossly assessing APD using intracardiac extracellular electrodes. The duration from the maximum negative slope of the unipolar "QRS" (activation) to the maximum positive slope of the "T-wave" (repolarization) correlates with the average of local action potential durations. I won't delve into the details of ARIs, but I'd just like to point out that you can't record ARIs from the atria because of their triangular-shaped action potentials.

[3] With constant conduction velocity the amplitude of the unipolar electrogram increases with the square of the distance between electrode and wave front, which means that the slope of the deflection doesn't remain fixed but gets progressively steeper.

[4] In reality both the positive and negative currents contribute to the potential field from all locations. Because amplitude falls with distance, whichever "pole" of the "dipole" is closer to the electrode has a greater impact on the net potential recorded.

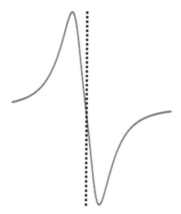

Figure 8.3 Unipolar electrogram. The unipolar signal records a positive deflection as a wave approaches the electrode and a negative deflection as it recedes. The rapid transition between positive and negative (max negative dV/dt) indicates the point at which the wave passes beneath the electrode.

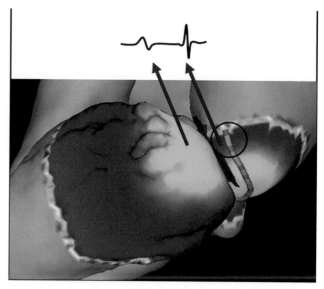

Figure 8.4 Near-field and far-field signals. Remote signals generate a smaller deflection on unipolar recordings than close signals. The coronary sinus typically sits over the atrium, and hence, on the CS catheter, atrial electrograms are sharper (and sometimes higher amplitude) than ventricular electrograms.

How can we tell whether we are looking at a wave that is passing immediately beneath our electrode or one that is far away?[5] In either case we see an upward deflection as the wave gets closer to our electrode and a negative deflection as the wave moves farther away. Can we distinguish near-field from far-field by looking at the amplitude of the electrogram? If it's true that amplitude diminishes with distance *and* that amplitude also diminishes as the current source is diminished – how can we tell whether we are looking at a large source from far away or a small source from nearby? The answer comes from combining the information derived from the *amplitude* with the information derived from the *slope*. Think about the geometrical relationship between wave front and electrode with a wave that is far-from vs. near-to the recording site (Figure 8.4). A far-field signal moves toward and then recedes from the electrode without ever getting close, and therefore such a signal never gets to a proximity where its slope is steep; i.e., far-field signals are more rounded than near-field (Figure 8.4). So, a small but "sharp" electrogram is probably from a small source close by (e.g., thin tissue or narrow fiber) rather than a large source far away.

So, we see an upward deflection as a wave approaches the electrode and a downward deflection as it leaves; interestingly, when the wave front is immediately beneath

the electrode the amplitude is zero. This is somewhat surprising when you think about it: it means that *when activation is immediately beneath the electrode you are completely blind to its presence.* The explanation is that the positive and negative portions of the dipole are equidistant from the electrode and completely cancel each other. There is an abrupt transition from a positive to a negative deflection as a wave passes our electrode; we generally interpret the maximum negative deflection – the transition from positive (approaching) to negative (receding) – as the **local activation time** (Figure 8.3).

While we can identify the time when the wave *front* passes beneath our electrode, we *cannot* tell when the trailing edge of repolarization passes by. This is unfortunate because, as we discussed at length in Chapter 4, wave length (the distance between the leading and trailing edge of activation) is a very important component of arrhythmogenicity. Why can't we see the repolarization wave? Remember we are measuring local potential, which is proportional to source current, which in turn is proportional to the voltage gradient. At the leading edge of depolarization there is a large voltage gradient over a short distance (between excited cells and adjacent unexcited cells). This produces a large current and hence a large potential. Because action potentials are

---

[5] Imagine watching a car pass by as you watch from (1) the side of the road (near-field) or (2) the middle of a field by the side of the road (far-field); in both cases the car gets closer as it approaches the part of the road nearest you and then gets farther away.

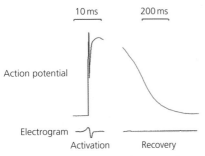

Figure 8.5 Intracardiac electrograms – activation and recovery. Analogous to EKG recordings, the intracardiac electrogram manifests a deflection as an activation wave front passes the electrodes but nothing when the repolarization wave passes.

shaped more like a triangle than a rectangle the gradient is much larger at the depolarizing wave than at the repolarizing wave. Hence repolarization produces a much lower amplitude and longer-lasting deflection, while depolarization produces a larger and shorter deflection (Figure 8.5). The intracardiac "T wave" is essentially lost, as it is close to the level of noise.

From the perspective of a unipolar electrode the direction from which a wave approaches is irrelevant; if a wave is approaching it generates a deflection. Soon we will see that the same cannot be said for bipolar electrograms; their amplitude is *direction-dependent*. A wave generates a positive deflection as it approaches the electrode and a negative deflection as it recedes. This can be used to identify the site of **earliest activation** (e.g., source of a focal tachycardia or insertion site of an accessory pathway). When you record from the site of earliest activation there is no positive deflection; the wave is always receding. Thus a "QS" complex suggests the site of earliest activation (Figure 8.6).

Bipolar electrograms

Bipolar electrograms are recorded when both electrodes are in the heart. Because electrograms reflect the *difference* between the signals recorded on each electrode (anode and cathode), that portion of the signal that is generated by a current from far away looks relatively similar to both electrodes and is therefore subtracted from the bipolar signal. As the current source gets closer to the electrodes the potential field it produces on each electrode (unipolar electrogram) begins to look less and

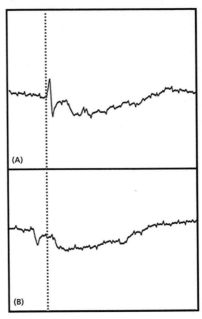

Figure 8.6 Unipolar morphology and site of earliest activation. (A) As a wave approaches the electrode there is a positive deflection on the unipolar tracing. (B) If the wave originates *at* the electrode, there is no positive deflection (the wave is never approaching the electrode). Note, if we are recording from the site where activation originates then not only will there be a QS morphology to the unipolar electrogram, but that site should be the earliest activation site.

less similar (see Chapter 7, Figure 7.2); hence the signal is not entirely subtracted away.[6] For this reason bipolar electrodes have higher spatial resolution than unipolar electrodes.

The morphology of a bipolar signal varies depending upon the direction from which a wave approaches the electrodes. The signal is maximal when the direction of the wave front is parallel to a line co-axial with the electrodes (Figure 8.7; see also Figure 7.5). It is minimal when the direction of the wave front is perpendicular to the inter-electrode axis. The morphology of the electrogram (RSR vs. QRS) depends upon whether the wave approaches from the cathode or anode side of the bipolar pair. Amongst other things, this can be useful information when a wave front arises from between two

---

[6] If you and I are looking at a tree on the top of a hill in the distance, it looks roughly the same to each of us. If you subtracted what I see from what you see we would see nothing (far-field subtraction). If, on the other hand, we were both looking at something that is between the two of us, it would look very different to each of us and hence *that* image wouldn't be subtracted away (near-field signal is not lost with bipolar recording).

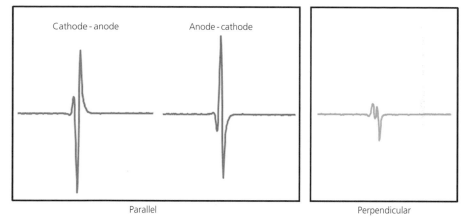

Figure 8.7 Bipolar electrogram morphology and wave direction. The bipolar electrogram is the result of subtracting one unipolar from the other. When the wave front travels *parallel* with the long axis between the electrodes both unipolar electrograms look the same *but are offset in time*. When the wave front is *perpendicular* to the long axis between the electrodes both unipolar electrograms look the same *and are superimposed in time*, so the difference is zero. In practice the wave front is never precisely symmetric, and therefore the perpendicular electrogram isn't zero. If the bipolar electrodes are parallel but lined up in the opposite direction (cathode and then anode) the electrogram morphology will be inverted.

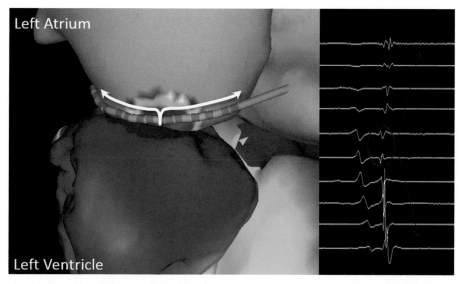

Figure 8.8 Bipolar electrogram morphology and site of earliest activation. When a wave spreads from between two bipolar electrode pairs their electrogram morphologies are opposite.

bipolar pairs; in this case the respective electrograms ought to have inverse morphology (Figure 8.8).

The improved spatial resolution of bipolar recordings is particularly important when mapping to identify an ablation target. For the purposes of *efficacy* one would like high resolution: a recording region smaller than the size of an RF lesion (that way, if you *see* it, you'll *kill* it). This does have *safety* consequences, because it also means that *just because you can't see it doesn't mean that you won't kill it*. For example, when mapping in the proximity of the His bundle one would not want a recording resolution that is smaller than the lesion size.

It can be quite helpful to record both unipolar and bipolar signals *simultaneously*. This allows both high resolution (bipolar) for efficacy and low resolution (unipolar) for safety. There is an additional advantage to recording unipolar and bipolar signals simultaneously from your ablation catheter: it allows you to determine whether a particular discrete signal is arising from the cathode or the anode. This matters, because while we

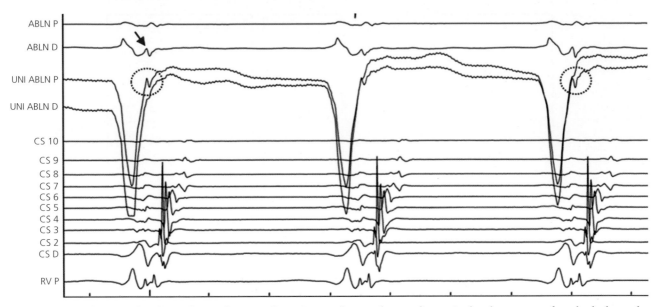

Figure 8.9 Simultaneous bipolar and unipolar recordings. By simultaneously recording unipolar electrograms from both electrodes that comprise a bipolar signal, one can discern whether the bipolar deflection arises due to activation at the tip or the ring electrode. On the first complex there is signal on the bipolar (ABLN D – red arrow); examination of the unipolar electrograms recorded from the ring (UNI ABLN P) and the tip (UNI ABLN D) electrodes indicates that the signal arises from beneath the ring electrode (red circle). When the catheter is pulled towards the ring electrode (second to third complexes) so that the tip ends up where the ring started, the signal can be seen to arise from beneath the tip (blue circle).

"map bipolar" we "ablate unipolar" – RF is only delivered via the tip electrode. An example of this can be seen with mapping of accessory pathways (AP). If there is an AP potential seen on one electrode but not the other, there will be a deflection on the bipolar electrogram (if it were on both electrodes it would be subtracted out and there would be no deflection on the bipolar). Thus the mere presence of a spike on the bipolar electrogram does not specifically indicate *which* electrode is above the source generating that spike. If the AP is beneath the ring electrode one simply needs to pull the catheter (moving the tip towards the ring) until the spike is on the unipolar electrogram recorded from the tip (Figure 8.9).

Discerning earliest activation

The site of earliest activation (EA) can indicate either the location of a focal rhythm or the insertion site from one tissue into another (e.g., where an accessory pathway inserts into the ventricle). "Earliest" refers to the timing of one site relative to all others. We therefore look at the local activation time and ask whether that time is earlier than the rest of the tissue. We can do this by moving a catheter around, assessing local activation time; it will get earlier as we move it towards the site of EA. Once we've reached the earliest site, the activation timing will get later when moving the catheter in any direction. Mapping for EA with a "roving" catheter employs comparison of the near-field (local) activation time from site to site. We can also compare the local activation time (LAT) to the earliest far-field timing. The surface EKG has such poor spatial resolution that it "sees" activation of the entire heart. You can compare LAT with earliest global activity. Clearly if LAT is *after* the earliest global excitation then the electrode cannot be at the site of EA.

What if LAT is equal to the earliest global timing? This likely does *not* indicate that you are at the EA site either. Consider what must happen for a deflection to appear on the surface EKG. When the "first cells" are excited they generate a potential field too small to be detected from the body surface. As the resultant wave propagates, the number of excited cells grows, ultimately reaching a source size large enough to cause a deflection on the body surface. *That* is the timing indicated by the "earliest activation" on the EKG. Therefore we anticipate that the true EA is *before* the earliest seen from the body surface. When we simultaneously record from our electrodes in both the unipolar and bipolar configurations we can see both local activation (higher-resolution bipolar) and global activation (lower-resolution unipolar). When the electrode is *not* at the site of earliest activation: the presence of the initial slow upward deflection tell us that we are not at EA,[7] *and* it tells us "what time we have to beat." The site of earliest activation must be as early as (or earlier than) the timing of the earliest far-field deflection.

General considerations

In practice it is common that there isn't just one wave/one tissue generating a deflection but several superimposed sources/deflections resulting in complex electrograms (see *Mapping accessory pathways* in Chapter 9). A very common example is the electrograms recorded from electrodes in the coronary sinus. These electrodes are close enough to the left atrium, left ventricle, and coronary sinus musculature that each generates deflections on the electrogram. In order to deduce macroscopic propagation it is frequently important to determine which deflections correlate with activation of which tissue. This raises the issue of multi-component electrograms. If you see an electrogram with more than one deflection it means that there is more than one discrete current source. In practice this means either a single group of cells being activated multiple times (temporal variability) or separate bundles of cells being independently activated[8] at slightly different times (spatiotemporal variability) (see *Spatial resolution*, Chapter 7). The simplest example of this is a "double potential" (Figure 8.10).

Double potentials basically tell you that two electrically separated groups of cells were activated.[9] In order to have a double potential these cells must be activated at slightly different times. In order for them to be activated separately there must be electrical separation between

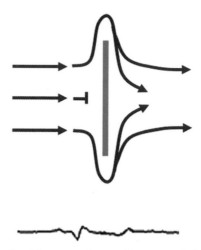

Figure 8.10 Double potentials. Double potentials (bottom) are seen when there are two separate activations of cells in the electrode recording region. The cartoon (top) depicts a classic scenario where one side of a linear scar and then the other is activated.

these groups of cells ... i.e., local block. This is easily appreciated along the annulus where A and V are in close proximity but (locally) electrically disconnected. It can also occur within the atria or ventricles at sites of local block, for example with a long narrow scar (e.g., surgical incision) or functional obstacle (e.g., the crista terminalis). Finally, during ablation, where cells beneath the electrode are destroyed, one often sees the emergence of a double potential as the ablation results in separation between the cells on either side of the lesion; activation now has to spread around the ablation lesion (Figure 8.11).

Once you've identified a double potential you can watch how the electrogram changes as you move your catheter. Moving to one side or the other of a line of block (perpendicular to the block) reveals a single potential with either the "early" or the "late" timing. Moving along the length of the line reveals a persistent double potential. As you approach the end of the line the two potentials get closer and closer in timing, ultimately merging into a single potential (Figure 8.12). This is a typical way to search (map) for a "hole" through an ablation line.

Mapping often requires the identification of very small signals. This can be problematic, particularly if there is significant "noise" obscuring the baseline. Interestingly, you can actually identify a signal that is "smaller than the noise." How? As with all attempts at

---

[7] At the site of earliest activation the wave is always receding (never approaching) the electrode, and hence there is no upward deflection on the unipolar electrogram.

[8] within the recording region of the electrode.

[9] If the time between potentials is short it is unlikely that the deflections represent two waves sequentially exciting *all* the cells in the electrode's recording region (i.e., two beats).

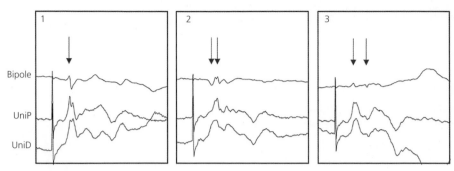

Figure 8.11 Lesion assessment using electrograms. (1) At the onset of RF there is a single potential (arrow). (2) As cells beneath the electrode become unexcitable the electrogram splits into two deflections (arrows) (reflecting activation at the near and far side of the electrode as seen from the activation wave). (3) As the lesion grows the splitting becomes more pronounced.

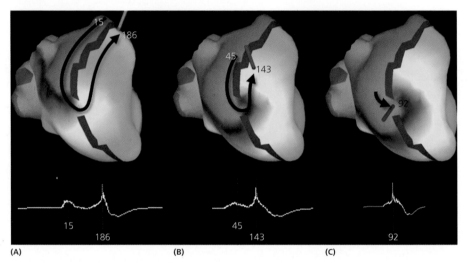

Figure 8.12 Double potentials around a line of block. Simulation of conduction (activation wave indicated by colored tissue; black arrows indicate direction of activation) around a line of block (dark gray) in the RA free wall. Activation travels down the left side of the linear scar and then up the right side. Therefore, (A) with the catheter placed superiorly and to the right of the line it records a far-field early electrogram (15 ms) and a late near-field electrogram (186 ms). (B) As the catheter is moved inferiorly, closer to the "hole" in the line of block, it records a later (45 ms) far-field signal and an earlier near-field signal (143 ms). Finally, (C) where propagation gets through the linear scar, the electrogram is no longer double; the near-field timing is earliest (92 ms).

differentiation, we look for something that is true about the signal but not true about the noise. If the signal is large and the noise is small we can use amplitude to distinguish signal from noise. This won't work when the signal-to-noise ratio is low. There is another difference that we can capitalize upon, however: noise is often random[10] (in time) while signal is periodic. A repetitive (periodic) alteration in the noise identifies a "real" signal (sometimes a larger signal, sometimes just a different shape, depending on when the signal falls relative to the largest deflection of the noise).

When looking for a small signal, it is very helpful to know where to look (not just *where* in the heart but also *when* in the electrogram). A good example is mapping to identify a "hole" through a scar: we know that the timing of conduction *through* the hole must occur after activation on one side and before activation on the other (Figure 8.12). Therefore we know at what timing we expect to find a signal.

There is a relationship between the spatial resolution of a catheter and its ability to identify small signals. Imagine a small discrete fiber conducting electricity through a large expanse of electrically silent scar (Figure 8.13). A large electrode may be blind to this fiber due to superposition (see Chapter 7). A large

---

[10] Or 60 Hz (due to AC currents in the EP lab).

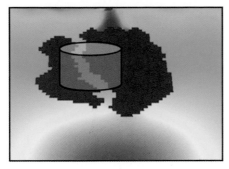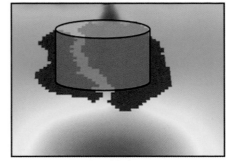

Figure 8.13 Spatial resolution and diseased tissue. It is not uncommon to find that no electrograms are recorded when mapping from an area of diseased tissue, despite the fact that propagation around the diseased area indicates that electricity is passing through it. This can occur when small channels of excitable cells pass through the diseased area. Smaller electrodes are more likely to detect a discernible signal due to a more favorable ratio of signal-generating tissue to quiescent tissue within their recording region.

electrode has a lot of surface area that is positioned over silent tissue (these regions contribute "zero" to the electrogram). Only a small portion of the electrode's surface sits over electrically active tissue. Because there can be no potential gradient on a conductor (electrode), the electrogram is an average of all the potentials that *would be* recorded at each site on the electrode (if it were not a conductor). Since a large number of "0s" are being averaged with only a few "1s" the actual deflection is very small (close to zero).[11] Consider, on the other hand, a small electrode. A greater percentage of the electrode's surface is over electrically active tissue compared with the large electrode (Figure 8.13); more "1s" relative to "0s" averages out to a *larger* signal.

Summary

- EKG vs. electrogram: the EKG offers global information about cardiac activity (its leads are approximately equidistant from all heart cells). Intracardiac electrograms offer improved spatial resolution because their position in the heart makes them closer to some cells than to others.
- The QRS is larger and sharper than the T wave because the voltage gradient and hence current

amplitude is larger during depolarization than during repolarization.
- Intracardiac electrograms indicate the leading edge of excitation and are essentially blind to the trailing edge of repolarization – because depolarization produces a larger voltage gradient (and hence current) over a short time interval while repolarization produces a small gradient (current) over a long time interval.
- Unipolar electrogram: grows as a wave approaches; has zero amplitude when the wave is directly beneath the electrode; transitions to a negative deflection as the wave passes the electrode; diminishes in amplitude as the wave recedes.
- The slope of the electrogram (dV/dt) relates to the proximity of the source current to the electrode (near-field signals are sharp; far-field signals are rounded).
- Local activation time (LAT): is the maximum negative deflection on the unipolar electrogram.
- The unipolar electrogram is entirely negative at the site of focal activation.
- Bipolar electrograms are the difference in potential between two electrodes. Distant signals "look" largely the same to both electrodes of the bipole while near signals look very different. As a result, bipolar recordings effectively "filter out" far-field signal.
- Contact bipolar electrogram amplitude is direction-dependent.
- Double potentials indicate local conduction block.
- One of the best ways to identify small signals is to know when (timing within the electrogram) to look for them.

---

[11] By this I mean that each portion of the electrode that sits on top of scar is contributing zero to the net potential averaged over the entire electrode surface. If most of the electrode sits over scar then only a small portion is contributing a non-zero signal to the average and hence the size of the electrogram is small.

9

Differential diagnostic pacing maneuvers

The purpose of this chapter is to introduce the principles of differential diagnostic pacing rather than to provide a recipe for how to approach every situation in which you may find yourself. The ideas that we make use of during differential diagnostic pacing are some of the most elegant in EP. You can use logic, along with a careful assessment of what you are told by your data (and what is merely suggested) to work through and figure out an enormous range of clinical cases.

At the outset there are two pieces of advice I can offer to the neophyte electrophysiologist. First, understand and remember that EP is waves of activation propagating through real 3D tissue – not squiggly lines on your monitor. If you always picture these waves as you try to discern what is "going on" and think of the electrograms simply as a small window into those waves as they traverse beneath your electrodes, you will fare much better. EP happens to occur in the "language" of electrograms; like learning any language, once you are fluent you no longer see letters on a page or electrograms on a screen but are taken to a world composed of the meaning of those symbols. Second, because we are looking only at a tiny fraction of the heart (beneath our electrodes), more than one activation pattern can produce the same electrogram sequence; the purpose of differential diagnostic pacing is to distinguish between these possibilities. Finally, at all times we seek a pacing site, sequence, or timing so as to maximize the difference between the possibilities.

Differential diagnosis of narrow complex tachycardia

When we observe a narrow complex tachycardia (NCT) we know one thing for sure: depolarization of the ventricles is via the His–Purkinje system (HPS). We know this because HPS conduction is *how* the complex gets narrow. Narrow means that the time between depolarization of the first and the last ventricular cell is less than 120 ms. If you were to stimulate the ventricle (with a PVC or a paced beat) sequential conduction across both chambers would take longer than 120 ms. The conduction distance divided by the conduction velocity equals the conduction time. The magic way that we can depolarize the entirety of the ventricles in less time than that required to propagate across them is that we depolarize multiple sites *in parallel* (see Video 9.1). The HPS is like an upside-down tree. The trunk is the His bundle, which then divides into an enormous number of branches. These form electrical connections with myocytes across the right and left ventricles. The result of parallel conduction is that propagation *isn't* spreading from cell to cell across the entire ventricles.

Simply knowing that ventricular activation is over the HPS is insufficient information to determine the rhythm. When we speak of diagnosing an arrhythmia, what we really mean is determining what *drives* that rhythm; in the parlance of cause and effect, the driver refers to that thing, the removal of which results in termination of the rhythm.

Understanding Clinical Cardiac Electrophysiology: A Conceptually Guided Approach, First Edition. Peter Spector.
© 2016 John Wiley & Sons, Inc. Published 2016 by John Wiley & Sons, Inc.
Companion website: www.wiley.com/go/spector/cardiac_electrophysiology

The differential diagnosis of NCT includes atrial tachycardia (AT), AV nodal reentrant tachycardia (AVNRT), and AV reciprocating tachycardia (AVRT); all of these conduct to the ventricles via the HPS. So we seek something that *differs* between these rhythms and then we look for the presence of that thing. AT and AVNRT do not include the HPS or ventricles in their arrhythmia *circuit*; only in AVRT are parts of the HPS and ventricles "in" the circuit. So our first step is to determine whether the ventricles can be dissociated from the rhythm. The idea is that AVRT is a macro-reentrant circuit. All the elements within a circuit are activated *in series*, i.e., activation of each site leads to activation of the next. The importance of this fact is that one cannot advance the timing of one element of a circuit without advancing all subsequent elements. "Advance," in this context, means cause-to-occur-earlier than it would due to the arrhythmia itself. It turns out that a tremendous amount can be discerned simply by differentiating between **serial and parallel conduction**. Serial conduction implies causation, e.g., conduction from the proximal to the distal His. Parallel conduction does *not* imply causation, e.g., activation of the right and left bundles from the His; both are caused by His activation but neither causes the other.

It is easy to understand this if you consider the following analogy. Imagine a rope with two knots. If you pull on the rope you cannot move the first knot without also moving the second knot; they are *in series*. Consider instead two ropes (side by side) each with a knot. In this case pulling on one of the ropes moves one of the knots but not the other; these knots are *in parallel*.

Step 1: Deliver PVCs

In the setting of NCT our first step is to determine whether the His (H) and ventricles (V) are in the circuit. If they are, you cannot advance the timing of V (or H) without advancing the timing of the subsequent atrial activation (A). We test this by pacing from the V during supraventricular tachycardia (SVT) at a time when the His is refractory. The importance of this particular timing is that if the His is refractory and you *can* advance the timing of the subsequent A *from the V* there must be an alternative way to get from V to A (in addition to the His/AV node (AVN)) (Figure 9.1).[1]

---

[1] By delivering a "late" PVC (during His refractoriness) the paced wave will collide with the antegrade SVT wave somewhere in the V or HPS (depending upon relative timing) and thus cannot get to the A via retrograde node.

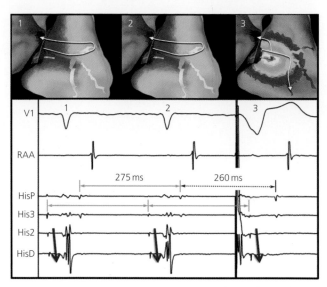

Figure 9.1 Late PVCs during narrow complex tachycardia. His-refractory PVC advances A, proving the existence of an accessory pathway. Note antegrade His deflections after pacing spike (red arrows). The PVC precedes His activation, so why isn't the His activated retrograde?

So, **a "late" premature ventricular contraction (PVC) that advances A** indicates the *presence* of an accessory pathway (AP), but this information alone is insufficient to determine whether that pathway is in the tachycardia circuit. For that, we need to look at more than just the timing of atrial activation. The basic situation with the differential diagnosis of NCT is that while we can see *what* the atrial activation sequence is we don't know what *causes* that sequence (i.e., is it retrograde AP, retrograde AVN, or AT?). When we advance A with a PVC we *do* know what caused *that* A (retrograde AP conduction), *and* we know what its activation sequence is. So now we can compare the activation sequence following the PVC with that during unperturbed SVT. If they are the same, then activation was going retrograde via the AP all along (i.e., the rhythm is AVRT); if activation is different, then the AP is simply a bystander (i.e., something else is causing atrial activation during SVT).

A late PVC that fails to advance A

There are two potential explanations for a late PVC that *doesn't* advance the timing of the subsequent A: (1) there is no causal relationship between V and A (i.e., not orthodromic reciprocating tachycardia, ORT), or (2) there *is* a causal relationship but our PVC has failed to identify it (i.e., there *is* an AP and the rhythm is ORT – see Video 9.2). It's easy to understand the first possibility: the PVC didn't advance A because His is refractory and there is no other way to get from V to A. The second possibility requires thinking a little more deeply. It is common to talk about (and think about) the atria and ventricles as if they were single, indivisible entities. In reality they comprise millions of cells that can act in a coordinated fashion, or not. Delivery of a PVC during SVT requires that the paced stimulus be delivered *before* the SVT wave reaches the paced site[2] (otherwise the tissue is refractory and pacing will not capture). If you capture, the tissue at the paced site is activated by the paced wave (not the tachycardia wave). When talking about V timing you must specify which portion of the "V" you are talking about. Portions of the ventricle are activated by fibers at the HPS–myocyte junctions, and then their neighbors are activated, etc. When you *also* pace, the cells at the pacing site are activated by the stimulus and then *their* neighbors are activated. As these two waves propagate, some regions of the ventricle will be activated by the paced wave and some by the antegrade HPS wave (depending upon each region's proximity to either of these waves). Only those portions of the V that are activated by the paced wave will be advanced. The *relevant* portion of the V (when performing differential diagnostic pacing to rule out AVRT) is the ventricular insertion site of the AP. Thus if you deliver a PVC at a site and time such that the paced wave doesn't reach the V insertion site of the AP, then the AP (and hence the A) will not be advanced. We don't know whether or not there is an AP until we've advanced activation *at the V insertion site of the AP*. But how do we know where the V insertion site is, if we don't even know if there *is* an AP? We have set out to answer the question "is this rhythm ORT?" By this we mean "is retrograde atrial activation due to conduction over and AP?" If the rhythm is ORT then the site of earliest atrial activation must be the atrial insertion site of the AP. Therefore we are testing for the presence (and use) of an AP whose atrial insertion site (if it exists) is the site of earliest atrial activation. The ventricular insertion site is therefore *in the vicinity* of the earliest A. I say "in the vicinity of" rather than "directly across the annulus from," because APs can be slanted such that the V insertion site is as much as a

centimeter away from the atrial insertion site. Therefore when ruling out ORT it is wise to deliver a PVC at a site and timing such that you advance V up to 1 cm from earliest A in each direction. If you still haven't advanced A, then retrograde conduction isn't via an AP (or there is decremental conduction over that AP which causes a delay that exactly offsets the amount of prematurity of the PVC).[3]

Why must an advanced V lead to an advanced A if the V and A are in the tachycardia circuit? This is actually an important concept which stems from the serial vs. parallel conduction story. Reentry implies a circuit, and each site in a circuit is activated *in series* by the site that precedes it.[4]

Step 2: Deliver earlier PVCs

With our late PVCs we have either made our diagnosis (no need for step 2) or we have determined that SVT *isn't* ORT. Thus, if we are still performing our EP study, we must now determine whether the rhythm is AVNRT or AT. As in any differential diagnostic maneuver, we are looking for a test that will indicate the difference between these two possibilities. If the rhythm is AVNRT then atrial activation is via the "AVN" – i.e., the fast AV nodal pathway (FP) or a slow AV nodal pathway (SP) – otherwise atrial activation arises from AT. As we've already noted, we know what atrial activation sequence *is* during SVT but we don't know what *caused* it. If we deliver PVCs early enough that we penetrate the HPS–AVN retrograde, thereby advancing A, then we know what the activation sequence is and we *do* know what caused it (retrograde "node"). We can now compare the activation sequence during SVT with that of the advanced A. If they are the same, then activation was

---

[2] This is what the P in PVC stands for: premature.

[3] This possibility can be eliminated by delivering PVCs at more than one coupling interval (the likelihood of each decrement exactly equaling each degree of prematurity is very, very low).

[4] In fact this isn't quite true. A reentry circuit can be thought of as a group of serial circuits *in parallel* (imagine the individual runners' lanes on a track; each lane is "*in series*" but adjacent lanes are "*in parallel*"). If there were only one cell at each site around the circuit then all cells would be *in series*. In reality there are rows of cells making up a wave front, and each *row* is activated by the preceding row. Thus rows are *in series*, but cells within a row are *in parallel*. I raise this confusing detail because the cells in a given row can be dissociated from one another. Therefore to advance the entire circuit one must advance the entire row. This becomes relevant when thinking about entrainment of the wide portion of a circuit (i.e., not a narrow isthmus).

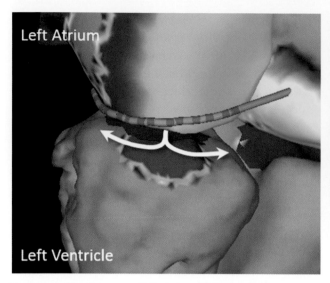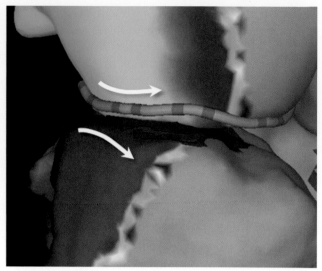

Figure 9.2 Continuous activity is insufficient to indicate accessory pathway site. With parallel conduction there can be many sites that have "continuous" activity; this is a non-specific finding and is inadequate to identify an ablation site.

"via the node" all along (AVNRT); if not, then the rhythm must be AT.[5]

Mapping accessory pathways

Before we turn to the question of how pacing can help to identify where to burn an AP, let's start by addressing appropriate targets for AP ablation. This may seem obvious but is a source of some misunderstanding. Luckily (or unfortunately) one can "get away with" using a non-specific target and still destroy the AP much of the time, but success rates are higher when more specific targets are used, and the associated clarification of EP concepts will improve your approach to all EP scenarios.

When asked "what is an appropriate target for AP ablation?" it is very common to hear "a site of continuous activation." The idea is that continuous activation indicates V leading directly to A and hence indicates an AP site. This, however, is based upon an assumption that V *causes* A. It is absolutely critical to assimilate the notion that just because one electrogram precedes another it does not necessarily mean that the earlier electrogram *caused* the later one ("association does not imply causation"). This is serial vs. parallel conduction again. If V and A are *in series* then V *does* cause A and continuous activity indicates the AP site. If V and A are activated *in parallel* then there is *no* causation and continuous activity is non-specific (Figure 9.2). We will explore this further below.

Appropriate targets for AP ablation are:
- the atrial insertion site
- the ventricular insertion site
- the AP itself

Identification of AP insertion sites

One truism about EP is that *earliest activation* indicates when/where propagation has *entered* a tissue (e.g., early V during pre-excitation or healthy tissue at the exit from a scar) but *late* activation does not indicate where activation *exits* a tissue. An obvious example of this is that atrial activation during sinus rhythm may enter the AVN well before the last atrial cells are activated somewhere in the left atrium. Thus a map of atrial activation will not indicate the location of the atrial insertion site of an AP during antegrade conduction; the ventricular activation sequence *will* indicate the AP's ventricular insertion site. A helpful analogy is looking for a hole in a balloon. The hole is too small to see directly, but if we place the balloon under water and look where the

---

[5] Technically you might argue that since there can be more than two AVN–atrial connections (one FP and several SPs) it is feasible that retrograde atrial activation during AVNRT could be via one SP but retrograde atrial activation of the advanced A is via a different SP. While this is possible, it would require that there be a portion of lower common pathway that is between the His and the "other" SP but isn't in the AVNRT circuit.

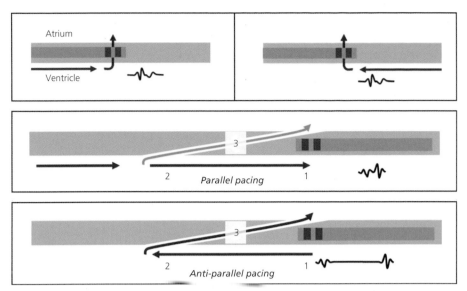

Figure 9.3 The significance of direction-dependence of VA timing. VA interval is only dependent upon the direction of ventricular activation (clockwise or counterclockwise) if there is a slanted accessory pathway. (Middle) With ventricular activation parallel to the AP slant, VA time is less than AP conduction time: V-at-V-insertion-site (2) to V-at-early-A (1) *minus* AP conduction time. (Bottom) In the "anti-parallel" direction (ventricular activation sequence and AP slant in opposite directions), VA time reflects the time from V-at-early-A (1) to V-at-V-insertion-site (2) *plus* AP conduction time (3).

bubbles arise from, we can infer where the hole is. Another example is finding a hole in a floor. If you watch water flow across the floor you may not be able to detect where the water is escaping; but if you watch the ceiling below it is obvious where the water is entering.

Identification of the AP itself

The ideal target for ablation is the AP itself, but it can be difficult to directly identify an AP potential. One problem is that the AP potential is small (compared to local atrial and ventricular electrograms). More importantly, activation of all three (A, AP, and V) can occur roughly at the same time such that their potentials are superimposed. The trick, then, is to separate the timing of A, AP, and V – but how?

Slanted accessory pathways

Fortunately, many APs are slanted (the atrial and ventricular insertion sites are not directly across the annulus from each other). We can take advantage of this slant to identify AP potentials. If you examine VA conduction time at the site of earliest atrial activation you will find an unusual thing: the VA time[6] *depends*

upon the direction of ventricular activation parallel to the annulus (Figure 9.3).

If the AP is perpendicular to the annulus then it shouldn't matter which direction the ventricular activation wave arrives from (Figure 9.3, top).[7] If the AP is slanted then the direction-dependence of VA timing makes perfect sense. Consider a slanted pathway with V-insertion to the left and A-insertion to the right. Let's first work through activation when a wave approaches the V-insertion site from the left (i.e., pacing is from the same side as the V-insertion site: this is called pacing in the "parallel" direction). The wave travels along the annulus left to right (Figure 9.3, middle). At the AP the wave divides into two, one portion continuing along the annulus and the other traveling up the AP. The V wave travels towards the site on the V side of the annulus directly across from earliest A *at the same time* as the AP wave travels up the AP towards the earliest A. Hence both waves arrive at the annular location of early A at roughly the same time. It is critical to distinguish the difference between V-at-early-A and the V-insertion site of the AP; with a slanted AP these are not the same

---

[6] In this context when we say "VA conduction time" we are specifically referring to the timing between the V and A *of the electrogram which records earliest atrial activation.*

[7] In reality subtle asymmetries in the fibers can result in different source–sink balance depending upon direction and hence variable conduction time. This has more of a theoretical than a practical impact.

location. VA at early A is measured between the V-at-early-A and A-at-early-A (i.e., from the electrode that records both potentials). Because activation is traveling *in parallel* towards both A-at-early-A and V-at-early-A, the VA time is short (and *isn't* the conduction time over the AP – it is the AP conduction time *minus* conduction time from the V-insertion site to V-at-early-A). Compare this with the situation when a wave approaches the AP from right to left along the annulus (Figure 9.3, bottom) (this is called pacing in the "anti-parallel" direction). The wave travels past V-at-early-A but doesn't activate A as it hasn't yet reached the AP. It then reaches the V at the V-insertion site. Here it divides into two, one part of the wave traveling up the AP and the other portion continuing along the annulus. Now VA time is long. Again, VA time isn't the AP conduction time – it is the time of conduction from the V-at-early-A to the V-insertion *plus* AP conduction time (V-at-V-insertion to A-at-A-insertion).

The slant explains the direction-dependence of VA time. It also provides an opportunity to maximize our chances of identifying an AP potential by separating the timing of V, AP, and A (by pacing from the "anti-parallel" direction). If we move our catheter along the annulus from V-at-early-A in the direction of the V-insertion site we can place our electrode at the mid-body of the AP. How do we know which direction the mid-body is relative to the A-insertion site? We know which direction the AP slants because of our differential pacing. The V-insertion site is in the direction from which VA timing was the shortest. If we pace from the "anti-parallel" direction, V (at our electrode site) occurs at a time when neither AP nor A is activated. Propagation then travels out of the view of our electrode, reaches the V-insertion site of the AP, and travels up the AP (beneath our electrode) inscribing an AP potential *after* local V and *before* local A. Activation then reaches A and travels in all directions, including back into our electrode's view.[8]

In the case of an AP that is perpendicular to the annulus, V-at-early-A and V-at-V-insertion of the AP are the same thing. VA timing is equal to AP conduction time, VA time is direction-independent, and the AP potential is obscured by V and A.

---

[8] Note that with a slant the mid-body of the AP is not at the site of earliest A (A is later).

We can draw several important conclusions from the preceding information:

- If the VA timing is direction-dependent there is (almost certainly) a slanted pathway.
- The direction from which VA timing is the *shortest* is the direction of the slant (e.g., if VA is shortest when V activation is from left to right, the V-insertion is to the left and the A-insertion is to the right).
- Thus one can determine if there is or is not a slant, and in which direction it slants, *without* identifying both AP insertion sites.

Taking advantage of a slant to identify an AP potential
So, if we have determined that there is a slanted AP and we've identified the direction of that slant, we can use this information to find the AP. Let's say, for example, that we know that the AP slants towards the right (V-insertion site rightward, A-insertion site leftward). Because we also know where the A-insertion site is (we've mapped earliest A) we now know in which direction we will find the AP (rightward). We can use this information: look for the AP slightly towards the right of the A-insertion site. We can also take advantage of the slant to separate the timing of A, V, and AP: we pace the ventricle in the anti-parallel direction (from left to right along the annulus). This maximizes our chances of finding an AP potential (we're looking in the right place, and we are moving the atrial and ventricular electrograms later and earlier (respectively) than the timing at which we expect to see the AP potential). This is an excellent example of "making your life easy." Use everything at your disposal to maximize your ability to succeed in the EP lab.

Para-Hisian pacing

Para-Hisian (PHis) pacing is designed to distinguish the *cause* of retrograde atrial activation: AVN or AP conduction. Leveraging once again the concepts of serial vs. parallel conduction, the goal of PHis pacing is to determine whether atrial activation time is dependent upon H-activation time (see Video 9.3). If one can dissociate H-timing from A-timing then one can conclude that H and A are not *in series*, i.e., H is not causing A, and therefore that there is an alternative means to get from V to A (i.e., an AP).

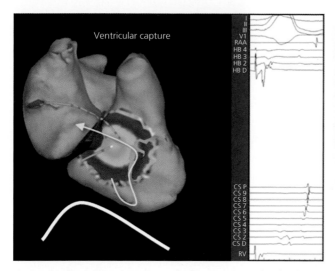
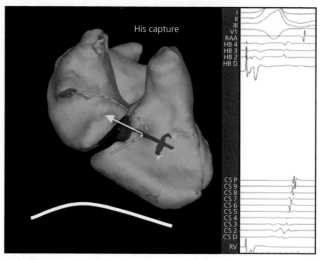

Figure 9.4 Para-Hisian pacing. The heart rests on the diaphragm and thus moves up and down with respiration; the catheter passes through a hole in the diaphragm and hence does not move with the heart. As a result the catheter can be placed such that it rests on the ventricle at expiration (left) and on the His bundle at inspiration (right).

Catheter placement

The goal is to determine whether retrograde A-timing and sequence are dependent upon the timing of H-activation. In order to determine whether A-timing is dependent upon H-timing we need to vary H-timing (and then see what happens to A). To achieve this, we compare pacing that captures H to pacing that doesn't capture H (V-only). This turns out to be easier to do than one might imagine. With a catheter placed in the anteroseptal RV it is close to the His bundle. As the patient breathes the heart (which sits on the diaphragm) moves up and down. The catheter (which passes through the diaphragm via the IVC) doesn't move up and down. The result is that the catheter alternately lies directly over H and then lies adjacent to H (on the V).

The His bundle is electrically insulated from the surrounding ventricular muscle. Thus when local V is captured activation does not propagate directly into the His; it must travel towards the apex, enter the right bundle branch (RBB) at the Purkinje–myocyte junction, propagate up the RBB, and *then* excite the H (only then does it produce retrograde atrial activation). In contrast, when the catheter directly captures H, activation proceeds straight to the A via the AVN and fast or slow pathway (Figure 9.4). What makes this pacing site so powerful in its capacity to differentiate is the discrepancy between retrograde conduction times with and without an accessory pathway (see Video 9.4).[9]

If H-capture advances A-timing

If A-timing is advanced with H-capture, this tells you that during the advanced beat atrial activation was due (at least in part) to H-capture (i.e., retrograde "node").[10] In direct analogy to PVCs delivered during SVT, we know what atrial activation sequence *is* during V-capture but we don't know what *causes* it. When A is advanced we know what the activation sequence is *and* what caused it. We can then compare A-activation sequence with and without H-capture. If they are the same, then activation was via the node all along (see Video 9.5). If they are different, then we know that there are two ways to get from V to A (see Video 9.6).[11]

If H-capture does not affect A-timing

If the timing of atrial activation is unchanged as H-timing is changed there are two possible explanations: (1) atrial activation is *not* via the HPS (i.e., it is via an AP), or (2) conduction *is* via the HPS but the shortened

---

[9] It is common to produce alternation between V-only capture and V-and-H capture. For the purposes of differentiating the retrograde conduction path it is sufficient that H is captured vs. not captured (regardless of whether V is captured as well).

[10] Retrograde atrial activation may be via the fast or slow pathways; to avoid laboriously writing this out I will refer to the combination of these possibilities simply as retrograde "node."

[11] While we now know that retrograde activation has two possible paths (there are two different activation sequences), we do not yet know whether H-capture is node only and V-capture is AP only, or if there is fusion during one or the other ... we only know that activation isn't the same under the two capture conditions.

coupling interval that results from H-capture (compared with V-capture) causes decremental conduction that increases conduction time by exactly the same amount that H-timing was advanced, such that atrial timing remains unchanged.[12]

Distinguishing between H-capture, V-capture, and both

In order to interpret PHis pacing it is critical to determine when you *have* and when you *haven't* captured H. There are several clues we can use to determine what we've captured on any given beat (H, V, or both). First, we can look at the QRS. During H-only capture the QRS should look identical to that during any supraventricular beat. The QRS is narrow (assuming normal HPS conduction). With V-only capture there is early activation of local V (immediately following the pacing stimulus) and the QRS is wide due to serial propagation outward from the pacing site. This typically means that the QRS begins early (direct V-capture) and ends late (absence of HPS conduction). With H- and V-capture the QRS begins early *and ends early as well*. The width of the QRS, as well as the timing of QRS initiation and QRS termination, all provide clues to the presence or absence of H- and V-capture. Our final clue is that with V-only capture H occurs late (that's the whole point). With H-capture it is common to *not* see an H deflection (H can be obscured by the pacing stimulus artifact).

Once we've determined *what* we've captured, we can begin the analysis of atrial timing and sequence. If the *timing* of A is dependent upon H-timing but its *sequence* is not, then retrograde conduction is not via an AP (i.e., retrograde node only). Note that I did not say "indicates the *absence* of an AP," only that there is absence *of conduction via* an AP. When there is an AP, the extent of atrial tissue that is activated via retrograde AP vs. retrograde node is entirely dependent upon the relative conduction times over the two paths to the A. This is directly analogous to pre-excitation, which is a race between antegrade AP and AVN/HPS conduction. It is not uncommon to see no retrograde atrial activation via a left lateral AP during either H-capture or RV-anteroseptal-capture (if conduction from the anteroseptum to the HPS and up through the node is faster than conduction across the left ventricle and up the AP).

Para-Hisian pacing 201[13]

Antegrade vs. retrograde His-dependence

I confess, I oversimplified above. The mere fact that atrial activation is H-capture-dependent does not actually definitively prove that retrograde conduction is via the node (even on the advanced beat). What?!

Below is an uncommon finding, but one that merits discussion, because it reminds us to remain on the lookout for *assumptions* that we may be making *without realizing it*. What possibility (other than retrograde node conduction) is there, if A-timing is dependent upon H-capture? A-timing may be dependent upon *antegrade* H-capture. The tracing in Figure 9.5 shows a left lateral AP in which A-timing, but not A-sequence, is H-capture-dependent. In this case, however, retrograde atrial activation is via the *AP* with and without H-capture. With V-only capture, conduction proceeds from the RV pacing site through the LV to the V-insertion site of the AP. With H-capture, V at the AP-insertion site is activated earlier due to rapid propagation through the left bundle branch, thereby advancing A without changing its sequence (in both cases there is no retrograde nodal conduction).

Eccentric activation

The last paragraph implies an important lesson for EP: beware of assumptions (especially those that you don't realize you've made). As we just saw, not all H-dependent retrograde activation is dependent upon *retrograde* node. Conversely, not all eccentric activation is retrograde AP. It is commonly assumed that the AVN–atrial pathways are all in the periseptal area, and hence that retrograde node produces a "concentric" atrial activation pattern (spreading across both atria from the septum). It is therefore common to conclude that all eccentric activation must be due to retrograde AP conduction. This is a risky assumption, as there can be left-sided SP fibers

---

[12] One could rule out this unlikely possibility by simply pacing the His even earlier.

[13] There are some subtleties to the interpretation of PHis pacing that we'll review below. These can be confusing. Make sure that you have a firm grasp of what we've discussed above before reading ahead.

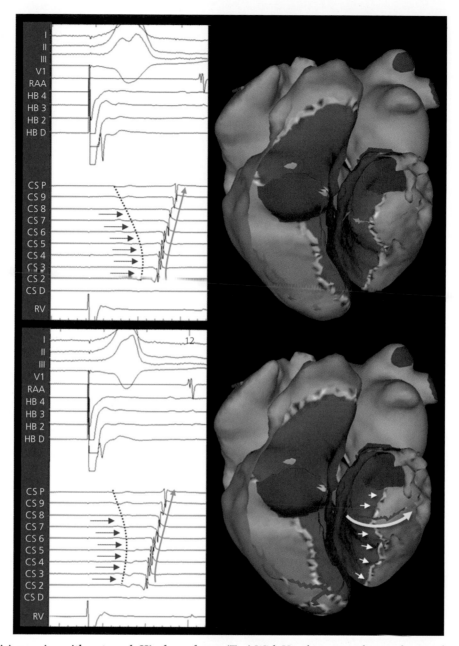

Figure 9.5 Para-Hisian pacing with *antegrade* His-dependence. (Top) With V-only capture, there is slow conduction from the RV anteroseptal base across to the ventricular insertion site of the left lateral AP. (Bottom) With V- *and* H-capture, the LV freewall (and therefore the V-insertion site of the AP) are excited *sooner* by propagation over the left bundle branch (yellow arrow) than they would be by the paced ventricular wave (white arrows). Note that the atrial activation sequence is the same for both beats, and the VA interval also remains the same (i.e., the A is advanced *because* the V is advanced).

that insert as far left as ~3:30–4:00 on the mitral annulus. Thus, we must examine not simply atrial activation sequence but also H-dependence. We've just finished demonstrating that it is possible to have eccentric activation that is H-dependent *and* due to an AP … so how can we ever distinguish retrograde AVN from retrograde AP? The first rule of differential diagnosis

is to identify a test which maximizes the differences between the diagnostic choices. What differs between retrograde node and retrograde AP, when both have a lateral insertion site? The answer remains the same as PHis pacing with concentric activation: ventricular activation adjacent to the site of early atrial activation. The local V at the site of early-A is *in series* with A in

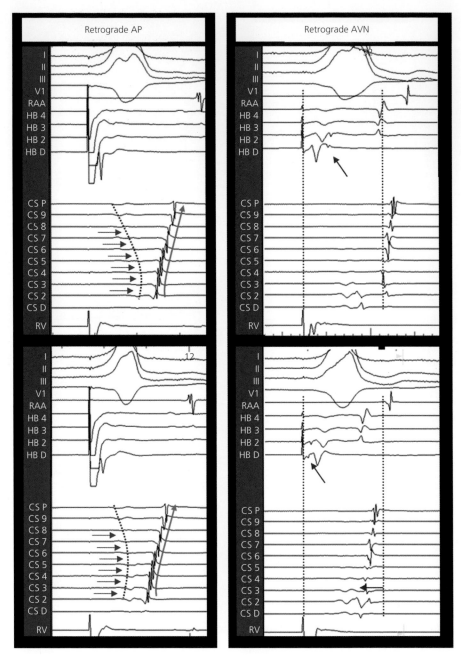

Figure 9.6 Eccentric activation does not always indicate an accessory pathway. Because we often think of the atrial insertion sites of the AVN as being in the center of the heart, it is not uncommon for electrophysiologists to assume that eccentric activation must be due to retrograde AP conduction. In the left panel we see that retrograde conduction timing, but not sequence, is His-dependent, suggesting that this is retrograde AVN conduction; but it is in fact AP conduction with antegrade His-dependence (Figure 9.5). In the right panel we also see that atrial activation timing, but not sequence, is His-dependent, and the atrial activation sequence is eccentric. In this case conduction *is* retrograde AVN. The clue that distinguishes the left tracings (retrograde AP – antegrade H-dependence) from the right tracings (retrograde AVN – retrograde H-dependence) is that *VA is fixed when activation is dependent upon V* (left) but varies when atrial activation is independent of V (right).

the case of an AP but *in parallel* with A in the case of retrograde node. Thus we can examine whether atrial timing and sequence are dependent upon the timing of local V *at early-A* (Figure 9.6).

In Figure 9.6 (right panel) you can see that the VA-at-early-A is *not* fixed, indicating that *this* V is not in series with the early-A, but the H is in series; hence this must be retrograde AVN conduction. In Figure 9.6 (left panel), VA *is* fixed at early-A (as is HA[14]), and therefore this is retrograde AP conduction.

Why is it that the timing from H to V-at-early-A is not fixed? With V-only capture, activation travels from the capture site through the ventricle to V-at-early-A; simultaneously (*in parallel*) activation travels to the nearest Purkinje–myocyte junction and up the bundle to the His. In the case of H-capture, activation travels from the His through the bundles to the V and then to V-at-early-A (*in series*). Thus with V-capture HV timing equals pace-site to H time *minus* pace-site to V-at-early-A; with H-capture HV timing is the time from H (the pace site) to V-at-early-A.[15]

Bundle branch block and para-Hisian pacing

The series of tracings in Figure 9.7 provides an excellent exercise in electrogram interpretation. In order to appropriately interpret these tracings you should determine (1) what has been captured (V, H, or both), (2) how conduction has occurred through the HPS, and *then* (3) how the atria are activated (retrograde).[16]

Entrainment

Entrainment refers to the capture of a reentrant rhythm by activation arising from a source other than the reentry (typically pacing). *Entrainment mapping* is the process whereby we attempt to determine whether the pacing site is "in" or "out" of a reentrant circuit, by examining the electrogram response to pacing. Before we launch directly into a "how-to" explanation of entrainment mapping, let's review the relevant wave–wave interactions.

In order to keep things clear in your mind it is particularly useful to think through what is happening with propagation at the level of the tissue before thinking about what a sampling of electrograms[17] will look like.

Pacemaker cells aside, cardiac cells basically wait passively until their neighbors are excited and then they become excited (and excite their neighbors). There can be more than one wave of propagation within the heart at any given time. What happens when there are two sources of excitation? Cardiac cells aren't picky; they'll be excited by whatever wave reaches them first. If there are two wave sources, excitation will propagate outward from each; these waves will collide somewhere in the tissue. Some areas of the tissue are excited by one of the waves and some by the other. How do cells decide which source to follow? They don't, they simply become excited whenever their neighbors are excited. Which wave drives which area of the heart is determined by which wave front reaches that area first. *When* a wave reaches a cell depends upon (a) the time the wave began to propagate, (b) the distance between the wave source (e.g., pacing site) and the cell in question, and (c) the conduction velocity. It is very much like the math word-problem "one car leaves Chicago heading eastbound ..."

Let's work through some scenarios. Imagine two pacing sites[18] stimulated at the same rate, and at the same time (i.e., not out of phase). Each will generate waves that collide somewhere in between the pacing sites. Some cells are "driven" by one pace site and some by the other. Because they are pacing at the same rate the waves will collide at the same location with each stimulus.

Now imagine instead of two pacing sites we have stable structural reentry generating one wave and pacing at a site remote from the reentry circuit generating the other wave (Figure 9.8B). If we pace at a rate faster than the tachycardia cycle length, each successive stimulus will occur earlier (relative to the tachycardia). Under these conditions the paced wave can travel farther towards the tachycardia circuit with each beat. The result is that the two waves will *collide progressively closer to the tachycardia circuit* (Figure 9.8B–D).[19]

---

[14] This tracing is an example of a common reality of para-Hisian pacing: sometimes we don't actually record a His potential. We can nonetheless deduce whether or not we are capturing His (as described in the text). Under these circumstances, it is reasonable to use the pacing spike to early-A timing as a surrogate for His-to-A timing. This is usually accurate to within 5–10 ms. You can see from Figure 9.7 (middle panel) that during "para-Hisian" pacing we typically capture RBB, resulting in a 5–10 ms delay between pacing spike and H.

[15] Bear in mind that in the presence of a slanted AP, the VA at early A is dependent upon the direction of ventricular activation. In this case as well, the variation in timing results from switching between serial and parallel conduction (see *Slanted accessory pathways*, above).

[16] The noteworthy findings are: (a) short spike to V, early-onset QRS and early end to QRS; (b) short spike to V, early-onset QRS but late end to QRS; (c) long spike to V with delayed-onset QRS, late-ending QRS.

[17] Recorded during that propagation.

[18] This discussion applies to any two sources of activation; it's just less awkward to say "pacing sites" than to say "wave sources" (this will apply to a pacing site and a reentry circuit as well).

[19] In fact the waves from any two drivers, at different rates, will collide progressively closer to the slower driver.

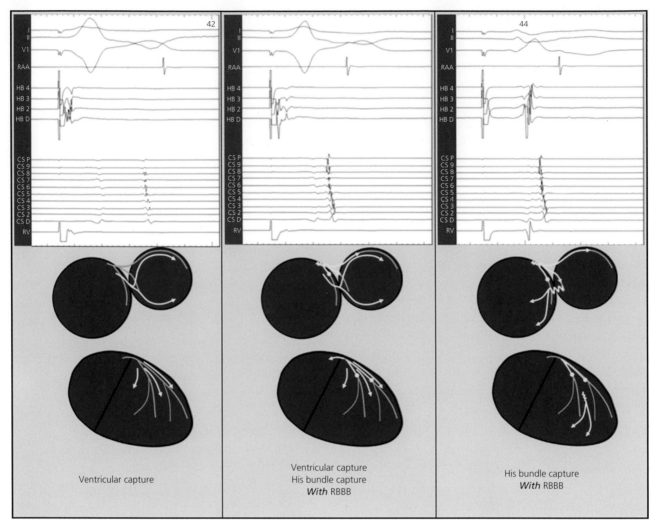

Figure 9.7 Para-Hisian pacing with right bundle branch block. The cartoons depict the heart in (top) LAO and (bottom) RAO projections. This series of three paced beats demonstrates the value of thinking through para-Hisian pacing systematically. In the first panel we see a wide QRS (not HPS conduction) that begins at the pacing stimulus, an early local V at the pace site (indicating V-capture), and a late A. In the second panel we see a slightly narrower QRS (the end of the QRS is earlier – due to H-capture), QRS onset is with the pacing stimulus, local V is early (V-capture), and A is earlier but with the same activation sequence. The first and second panels taken together indicate retrograde AVN conduction (atrial timing is dependent upon H-timing and sequence is not). In the third panel we see a wide QRS (starts late (not with stimulus) and ends late), there is not early V at the stimulus (no V-capture), in fact the local V is later than normal because of the RBBB (activation must spread from the LBB then through the septum), and atrial activation is early while the sequence is the same as panels 1 and 2. Here we've captured H only *and* there is right bundle branch block.

Ultimately the paced wave arrives at some part of the reentry circuit *before* the next reentry wave arrives. When the paced wave reaches a point in the circuit *earlier* than the preceding tachycardia wave, pacing is said to *capture* the circuit (Figure 9.8E). The paced wave splits at the structural circuit. One part travels in the direction that the tachycardia was traveling (the *orthodromic* wave) while the other travels in the direction opposite that in which the tachycardia was traveling

(the *antidromic* wave). The orthodromic wave (having stimulated the circuit before the next tachycardia beat arrives) *resets* the circuit. The antidromic wave (traveling the "wrong" way around the circuit) causes *fusion*. The antidromic wave collides with the *preceding* orthodromic wave part way around the circuit (Figure 9.9).

Once the paced wave has captured the circuit *there is only one source of excitation* in the tissue. All cells are now activated by the paced wave. The orthodromic and

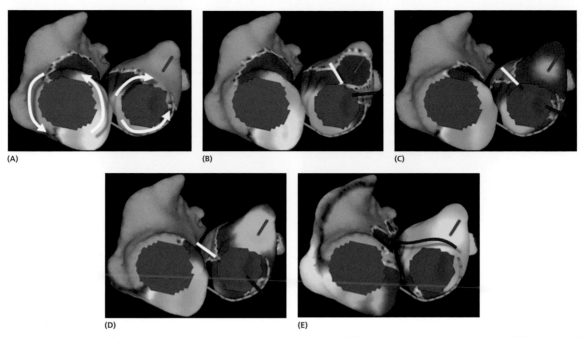

Figure 9.8 Entrainment with progressive fusion. (A) Counterclockwise atrial flutter (note that activation of the left atrium is both clockwise and counterclockwise around the mitral annulus). (B) Onset of pacing from the left atrium (far from circuit); the paced wave collides with the tachycardia waves. (B–D) As the paced beats fall progressively earlier relative to the tachycardia beats (pacing is faster) the paced and tachycardia waves collide progressively closer to the flutter circuit. (E) Once the paced wave arrives at the flutter circuit *earlier than* the flutter wave, we have captured the circuit. The entire heart is now activated *at the paced rate only* (there are no longer any sites excited at the tachycardia rate).

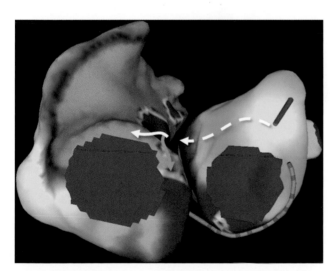

Figure 9.9 Antidromic and orthodromic waves. The paced wave crosses the left atrium (dashed white arrow) and excites the right atrium via the fossa. It then propagates in both directions around the tricuspid annulus. The clockwise (antidromic) wave (green arrow) soon collides with the previous paced capture beat. The counterclockwise beat (white arrow) travels along the same path (and in the same direction) that the tachycardia traveled.

antidromic portions of the paced wave arise at the same rate (the paced rate) and hence their collision site will remain fixed.

Pacing from outside the circuit

There are three different phases of activation when one paces during reentry (from outside of the reentry circuit).

Phase 1: The progressive fusion phase (as the paced wave collides progressively closer to the reentry circuit: see Video 9.7).

Phase 2: The entrainment or continuous resetting phase. This is often referred to as *constant fusion* (to distinguish it from progressive fusion). In reality it isn't truly fusion at all; remember, fusion refers to activation of tissue by *two separate* sources. It is nonetheless referred to as fusion because a portion of the tissue is activated in the same way during pacing as it was during reentry (the orthodromic wave) but another portion is activated *differently* (the antidromic wave).

Note that there is a different activation pattern if you start pacing *during* reentry vs. *before* reentry. The difference between pacing during reentry and pacing without reentry lies in the relative *sizes* of the anti- and orthodromic waves. As a result of this difference, the QRS morphology during pace mapping may be different from that during entrainment pacing. In the absence of ongoing reentry there is nothing to prevent the paced wave from traveling in the antidromic direction (there is no orthodromic reentry wave causing block of the antidromic wave (Figure 9.10). As a result the orthodromic and antidromic waves will travel equal distances[20] around the circuit and collide on the far side. The *asymmetry of reentry* (reentry circulates in only one direction around a circuit) *induces an asymmetry in the paced wave.*

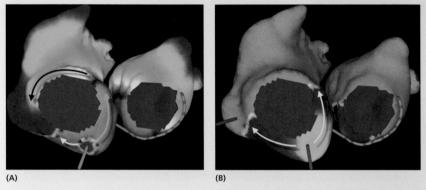

(A)   (B)

Figure 9.10 Entrainment pacing vs "straight" pacing. (A) Pacing from the CTI during flutter, the paced wave divides into a clockwise (yellow arrow – antidromic) and counterclockwise (green arrow – orthodromic) wave. The antidromic wave is shorter than the orthodromic wave (will be) because it runs into the previous paced orthodromic wave (black arrow). (B) When "straight" pacing (not during tachycardia) the ortho- and antidromic waves each travel unobstructed until they fuse at the far side of the annulus.

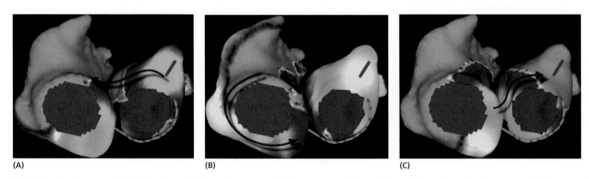

(A)   (B)   (C)

Figure 9.11 Pacing from outside the circuit. Once the pace site has captured the tachycardia and pacing has stopped, the paced wave must travel (A) to the circuit, (B) around the circuit, and (C) back to the pacing site. Therefore the post-pacing interval (PPI) is longer than the tachycardia cycle length (TCL) (during tachycardia, activation only has to travel around the circuit).

Phase 3: The post-pacing phase. Once pacing is stopped the antidromic portion of the final paced beat collides with the orthodromic portion of the *prior paced beat*; the orthodromic portion of the final paced beat propagates around the circuit, but this time there is no antidromic wave with which to collide and reentry begins anew. Amongst other places, this first (new) beat of reentry now propagates back to the pacing site (but in the opposite direction from that during pacing) (Figure 9.11). So, at the conclusion of pacing, propagation must travel *to* the circuit, *around* the circuit, and then *back* to the pacing site (see Video 9.8).

Pacing from inside the circuit

What happens if pacing begins *in* the reentry circuit? The paced wave will *immediately* capture the circuit. Just as before it will divide into anti- and orthodromic waves; the paced source now has control of the entire tissue. The antidromic wave collides with the last reentry

---

[20] "Distance" here is measured in conduction time (not millimeters), so actual distance depends upon conduction velocities.

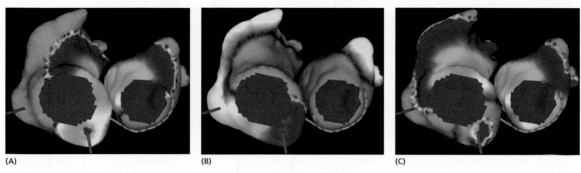

(A)   **(B)**   **(C)**

Figure 9.12 Pacing through the refractory period to capture the fully excitable gap. (A) This beat falls approximately halfway through the tachycardia cycle (the leading edge is at 11:30; pacing is at 5:30); the tissue is refractory and pacing will not capture locally. (B) Because the pace cycle length is less than the tachycardia cycle length, the tachycardia wave has progressed less far from the pace site on the next paced beat (3:30). (C) Eventually we pace *before* the tachycardia wave arrives at the pace site, and we capture locally. Because we are pacing inside the circuit we immediately capture the circuit.

wave; the orthodromic wave captures the remainder of the tissue. Importantly, **there is no progressive fusion**; the entire tissue is captured in the same way with each paced beat. When pacing *in the circuit* there is no phase 1 (progressive fusion) because there is *only one* driver/ source (pacing); so, however the wave splits, the site where *those* waves collide will be the same with every subsequent paced beat (Figure 9.10A). Phase 2 commences immediately, and the size of the antidromic wave is determined by how early the first beat is relative to tachycardia.

If pacing is initiated with a triggered beat (i.e., one specifically timed at the pace cycle length after a sensed beat at the paced site), then the cycle length between the last tachycardia beat and the first paced beat will be the same as the pace cycle length (PCL). If the timing of this first beat falls within the fully excitable gap (see *Reentry*, Chapter 4), it will propagate with the same conduction velocity as during tachycardia; therefore the post-pacing interval (PPI) will equal the tachycardia cycle length (TCL). If, however, the paced beat falls within the partially excitable gap, it will conduct at a *slower* conduction velocity than during tachycardia. The cycle length will remain the paced cycle length, but the conduction times will increase; therefore the PPI will be longer than the TCL (due to slower conduction velocity during pacing). Much of our interpretation of the response to pacing presupposes that the paced and tachycardia conduction velocities are the same. If propagation is slower with pacing, then we will *misinterpret* the PPI/TCL relationship as indicating we are pacing outside the circuit.

If the first paced beat falls in the absolute refractory period it will not capture (Figure 9.12A). Subsequent beats will fall progressively *earlier* relative to the tachycardia wave (Figure 9.12B). Once the paced beat is early enough it will occur *prior* to arrival of the tachycardia wave and can capture. At this point it is *most* likely to fall in the fully excitable gap (if there is one) (Figure 9.12C).

Interpreting entrainment pacing
Onset of pacing
With entrainment we are asking the question "is the pacing site inside the reentry circuit?" There are several clues that will allow us to answer this question. As we've just discussed, when we pace from *inside* the circuit we immediately capture the circuit; with pacing from *outside* the circuit there is progressive fusion prior to circuit capture. So, how can we tell when we've captured the circuit? Before we capture reentry there are two sources of excitation (reentry and pacing) *at different rates*. Thus, if examination of the electrograms shows that some sites are activated at the tachycardia rate and others at the pacing rate, then we haven't captured the circuit (Figure 9.13), so we are *outside* the circuit.

If all electrograms are at the paced cycle length then we *may* have captured the circuit. Remember that when we record electrograms we are only looking at a sampling of the heart's electrical activity. The absence of electrograms at the tachycardia rate could mean that the entire heart is activated at the paced rate, or that we are not recording electrograms from those areas at the tachycardia cycle length. So if we see some electrograms at the tachycardia rate we know that we are not pacing inside the circuit. If we see that all electrograms are

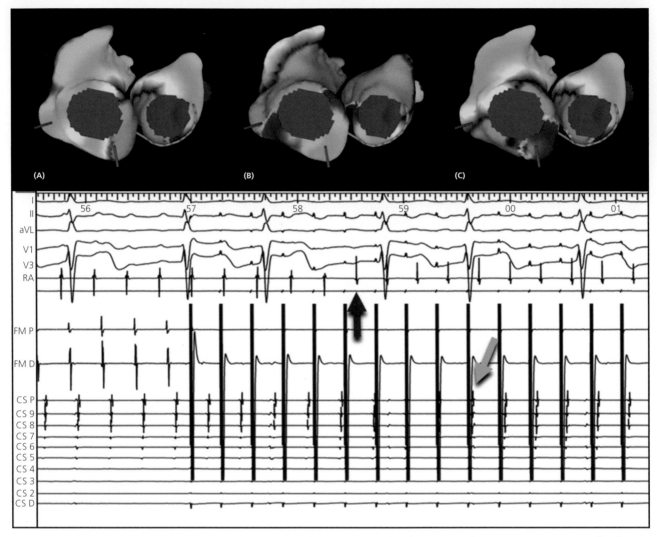

Figure 9.13 Electrograms at two rates indicate pacing outside the circuit. (A) Before pacing, the entire atria are activated at the tachycardia cycle length. (B) With pacing outside the circuit (this is clockwise left atrial flutter and we are pacing from the CTI) we capture the right atrial appendage (RA) on the sixth paced beat (red arrow) but the left atrium is still excited at the slower tachycardia cycle length (examine the CS electrograms: note that between the red and green arrows CS deflections are obscured by the pacing artifact). (C) Finally, by the tenth beat we have capture the circuit (CS is now at the paced rate). The fact that we can capture some areas while others are still slower means that we are not in the circuit.

immediately at the paced rate we *suspect* that we are inside the circuit. If we see that electrograms far away from our pacing site are immediately at the paced rate we are more confident that we are pacing inside the circuit (Figure 9.14).[21]

Analysis of electrograms acquired during pacing

If we have evidence that we have not immediately captured the circuit (progressive fusion,[22] different electrograms at different rates,[23] or progressive fusion on the surface EKG), then we know we are out of the circuit. Imagine that we haven't actually captured the entire heart but have captured all the sites where we have electrodes. If we see evidence of *progressive* fusion (e.g., on the EKG) we would know that we are not pacing inside the circuit.

---

[21] If we can only see recorded electrograms very close to our paced site we are less confident

[22] Progressive fusion indicates collision at different sites with successive beats; this means drivers at two rates, which cannot occur once you've captured the circuit.

[23] If we have different electrograms at different rates, by definition we have progressive fusion.

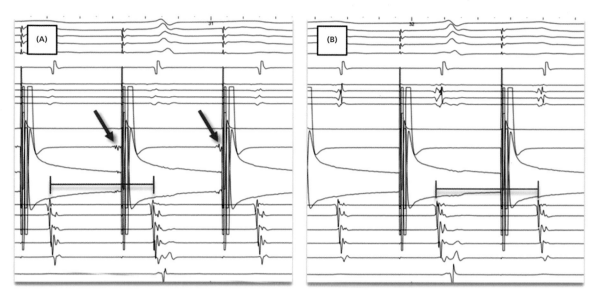

Figure 9.14 Interpreting entrainment during pacing. (A) Early in pacing we have not yet captured locally (we are pacing *after* local excitation – red arrows). (B) As soon as we capture the pace site we capture everything (everything we can see – the His, RA, and CS catheters). This indicates that we are pacing inside the circuit; there is no progressive fusion (which is the merging of two waves *at different rates*).

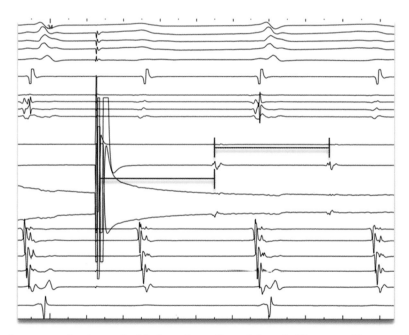

Figure 9.15 Comparing the post-pacing interval with the tachycardia cycle length. The interval between the last paced beat (spike) and the first return beat (local electrogram on paced electrode) is the post-pacing interval (PPI). The interval between the first return beat and the next beat is the tachycardia cycle length (TCL). When PPI = TCL we are pacing inside the circuit.

Analysis of electrograms acquired after pacing stops

Our final opportunity to analyze our electrograms is at the conclusion of pacing. If we are pacing inside the circuit, our last paced beat travels around the entire circuit and returns to the paced site. If the conduction velocity is the same during pacing and tachycardia, then the time required to return to the pacing site at cessation of pacing (the **post-pacing interval**, PPI) will equal the tachycardia cycle length (TCL) (Figure 9.15).[24]

---

[24] Conduction time equals conduction distance (the path length of the circuit) divided by conduction velocity.

Compare this with pacing from outside the circuit. The last paced beat must travel from the pacing site *to* the circuit, *around* the circuit, and then *back* to the paced site (Figure 9.11). Thus if we pace outside the circuit our PPI is longer than the TCL.[25] Note that our interpretation of the PPI *assumes* that the conduction velocity is the same during pacing and tachycardia. If conduction velocity is slower during pacing, the PPI will be longer than TCL *even if we are pacing in the circuit*. Practically speaking, this means that if the reentry circuit has no fully excitable gap we cannot properly interpret the PPI. This is one reason that it is beneficial to look for immediate capture (and the absence of progressive fusion). Finally, sometimes we terminate tachycardia with our pacing. In this case we cannot interpret the PPI but, again, we can examine the timing of capture and the presence of fusion.

Pacing from outside the circuit ... what next?

When we perform entrainment mapping we are trying to determine whether our pacing site is in or out of the tachycardia circuit. If we see that we are pacing outside the circuit, can we use the data acquired during pacing to decide where we should pace next? The answer can be found by considering what is happening when we pace outside the circuit. We know that the paced wave and the tachycardia wave collide progressively closer to the tachycardia circuit. We also know we can look at each electrogram and determine whether it is being driven by the paced wave or the reentry circuit simply by looking at the rate of that electrogram. Because the paced wave collides progressively closer to the circuit, electrograms will speed up to the paced rate *closer to the circuit* with each successive beat. The last sites to reach the pacing rate are in the circuit itself. Thus, the electrode whose electrogram reaches the pacing rate *last* is closest to (or in) the circuit. The next place to attempt entrainment is at (or beyond) *the last electrode captured by pacing*.

---

[25] Equal to the tachycardia cycle length *plus* twice the conduction time between the paced site and the circuit.

Summary

Differential diagnosis of narrow complex tachycardia (NCT)

- "Narrow" indicates conduction via the His–Purkinje system (parallel activation of ventricles).
- Differential diagnostic maneuvers very often leverage the differences between serial and parallel conduction.
- Differential diagnosis of NCT: atrial tachycardia (AT), AV nodal reentry tachycardia (AVNRT), orthodromic reciprocating tachycardia (ORT).
- Only ORT has ventricle in the circuit.
- His-refractory PVCs:
  ○ If they advance atrial activation then an accessory pathway is *present* (but not necessarily in the arrhythmia circuit).
  ○ If they advance atrial timing *and* the atrial activation sequence is the same, then the rhythm is ORT.
- Earlier PVCs:
  ○ When early PVCs advance His and atrial activation timing: is atrial activation sequence the same?
    – Yes: the rhythm is AVNRT.
    – No: the rhythm is AT.

Mapping accessory pathways

- Appropriate targets are early activation or an accessory pathway potential. Continuous ventricular and atrial electrograms are *not* an appropriate target.
- Slanted accessory pathways allow separation between atrial, ventricular, and accessory pathway electrograms (when pacing in the anti-parallel direction).

Para-Hisian pacing

- If atrial timing is dependent on His timing, but atrial sequence is not, then activation is retrograde node. If atrial timing is His-dependent, but atrial sequence varies with and without His capture, then an accessory pathway is present.
- If atrial activation timing and sequence are independent of His timing, then conduction is via an accessory pathway and not the node.
- His capture: the pacing spike is followed by a delay before local ventricular activation, there is a narrow QRS (late start, early finish).

- Ventricular capture: the pacing spike is immediately followed by local ventricular activation, there is a wide QRS (early start, late finish).
- His and ventricular capture: the pacing spike is followed by early ventricular activation, the QRS width is intermediate in duration (early start but also early finish).

Entrainment

- Answers the question "is the pacing site in the circuit?"
- Pacing outside the circuit:
  - Three phases:
    - Progressive fusion: collision progressively closer to circuit.
    - Entrainment/continuous resetting: orthodromic and antidromic waves; the entire tissue is activated at the paced rate.
    - Post-pacing phase: reentry resumes; the post-pacing interval (PPI) equals conduction time from the pace site to the circuit, around the circuit and back to the pace site: PPI > TCL.
- Pacing inside the circuit: immediately captures the circuit (the whole heart is immediately activated at the PCL). There is no progressive fusion. PPI = TCL.
- Interpretation:
  - Pacing onset: immediate capture? (Yes: in circuit).
  - During pacing: progressive fusion? (No: in circuit).
  - Post pacing: PPI = TCL? (Yes: in circuit).

10

Electro-anatomic mapping

There are two "types" of mapping: activation mapping and substrate mapping. We will discuss both.

Activation mapping

When we refer to electro-anatomic mapping (typically "mapping" for short) for the most part we mean activation mapping. There's more to it, but we'll get to that later in this chapter. In general, activation mapping is performed sequentially. Meaning that we aren't recording from multiple electrodes at the same time; instead we record at one site and then the next and the next. In order to perform sequential mapping we choose some fixed location as a reference and measure the timing of activation at various sites in the heart relative to the timing of activation at the reference site. Provided that (1) the rhythm is the same from beat to beat over the mapping period and that (2) the reference catheter doesn't move, the activation map created with sequential mapping will be the same as with single-beat (multi-site simultaneous) mapping. Regardless of whether we are creating a true single-beat map or a sequential map, we are only measuring electrograms at a sampling of locations; we are guessing about the timing of activation elsewhere (this is called interpolation). We must remain vigilant against misinterpretation due to interpolation.

Choosing a reference electrode/ electrogram

The accuracy of your map depends upon comparing all map points to the same reference timing. This means that the reference electrode must be in a physically stable position. In particular you want to avoid inadvertently moving the reference catheter with the mapping (sometimes called "roving") catheter. A good option for achieving reference catheter stability is to place it in the coronary sinus (CS). For one thing, the CS is a tube and hence less conducive to catheter movement then a chamber. Also, so long as you are not mapping within the CS it's pretty easy to avoid accidentally moving the reference catheter. It's not a bad idea to save a fluoroscopic image of the reference catheter position; later on, this can make it easier to decide if it has inadvertently been moved. The other requirement is that the reference electrogram be electrically stable. Even if the rhythm isn't varying it is possible to accidently compare local activation time at each map site to a different portion of the reference electrogram. This is particularly easy to do if the reference electrogram is biphasic; you must not sometimes use the first "hump" as a reference and at other times the second (Figure 10.1B). Because the CS catheter lies along the annulus it is not uncommon to record atrial and ventricular activity; it is critical to avoid annotating the A on some beats and the V on others (Figure 10.1C). Some people use a surface EKG lead as a reference. In general it is best to avoid this, as the ideal reference electrogram is a sharp signal that allows you to annotate the same part of the electrogram with each beat.

Choosing an annotation window

There are multiple ways to do this. I will not go through all of them or their relative advantages. Instead I will describe what we do in our lab and why. Provided we are mapping a rhythm that we believe may be reentry I will set the width of my annotation window to the tachycardia cycle length. This way there will be no place in the heart where you could find an activation time that doesn't

Understanding Clinical Cardiac Electrophysiology: A Conceptually Guided Approach, First Edition. Peter Spector.
© 2016 John Wiley & Sons, Inc. Published 2016 by John Wiley & Sons, Inc.
Companion website: www.wiley.com/go/spector/cardiac_electrophysiology

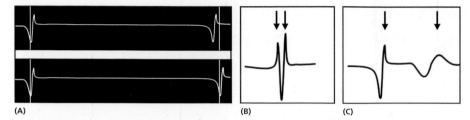

Figure 10.1 Annotation window. (A) If you set your annotation window from 0 to the tachycardia cycle length (TCL), then the second reference electrogram will fall directly on the annotation line when the TCL equals the annotation CL but will fall "off" the line during long or short cycles. Choose a reference signal that has a single discrete deflection. (B) If there are two "maxima," then annotate the minima. (C) If there is A and V, try to find a site where V is much less prominent.

fall within the window. The window is set relative to the reference electrogram. For example you could set a 300 ms window from 100 ms before the reference to 200 ms after. We prefer to set the window so it starts and ends on the reference electrogram (i.e., from 0 to 300 ms). Here's the rationale. It is all too common for reentrant rhythms to "wobble," meaning that the cycle length alternates by 5–15 ms or more. Under these circumstances you want to map only beats with the same cycle length. It can be difficult to notice that the distance between two electrograms has increased by 5–15 ms. If, however, you set your window to start and end with the reference electrogram there will be a line on both electrograms whenever the cycle length is 300 ms (Figure 10.1A). When the cycle length is longer or shorter the second electrogram will fall before or after the line. This difference is so easy to notice, you can detect it with your peripheral vision. For the same reason it is very easy to detect a change in the tachycardia cycle length.

The map colors

When we create a map we display color-coded activation times onto a 3D anatomic representation of the chamber being mapped. A scale is set up in which colors vary from the earliest portion *of the chosen annotation window* to the latest portion.[1] Thus colors reflect relative timing.

Double and fractionated potentials

The system can only assign one color (one local activation time) to a given site. As we discussed in Chapter 8, local conduction block can produce two local activation

times, i.e., a double potential (Figure 10.2A). The system requires that you choose one of those as the local activation time (LAT). How do you choose? To answer this we must discuss an important aspect of mapping: we are constructing a 3D picture of activation. To do this effectively it is very helpful to pay attention to the unfolding story the map tells *as you acquire data*. For example, as you move a catheter in the vicinity of a double potential you will see that in one direction the signal becomes single and "times with" the earlier potential, while in the opposite direction the electrogram is single and times with the later potential. You will likely also note that the double potentials exist along a line. It is easiest to interpret the map if you annotate the earlier hump when points are located slightly towards the direction that is earlier and annotate the later hump when points are located slightly towards the "late" direction. The same idea applies to fractionated signals. These can sometimes span 25–50% of the annotation window (Figure 10.2B). It helps to annotate at the time that is closest to the nearby times (and then mark the site with a tag that indicates local fractionation).

Sample density and interpolation

When you think about creating a map the idea is basically to recreate a color picture of activation timing throughout the heart. The heart is actually made up of millions of individual cells, each of which has an activation time. We can't, and don't want to, measure the activation timing at millions of sites. Instead we would like to measure activation at a much smaller number of sites and use that information to decide what the activation timing is at the sites we haven't measured. With this in mind, how do we decide *where* to "take points" and *how many* to take? We can look at the information we've acquired and try to decide where we need more.

---

[1] Note the difference between earliest in the annotation window (entirely dependent upon the window you select) and earliest in the heart (independent of your window choice). So, don't assume that "early" in the color scheme means early in the tissue.

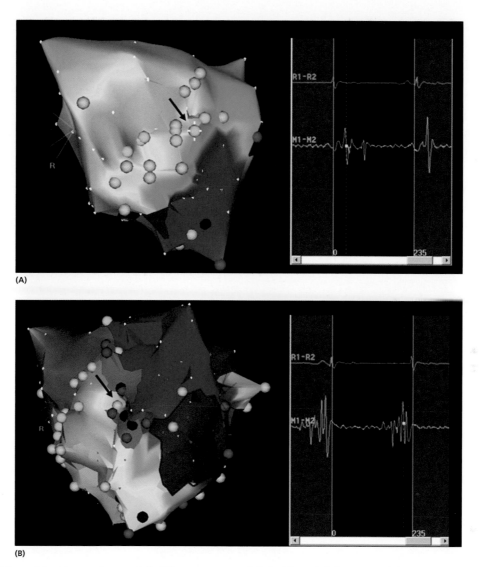

Figure 10.2 Double and fractionated potentials. When annotating (A) double or (B) fractionated electrograms it is helpful to choose a time that fits with the local context of the map. It can also be helpful to indicate the type of potential with an annotation tag (colored dots here – double (blue) or fractionated (pink)).

The "trick" is to update your interpretation of the map as you add points. This may not be natural for you. When I started mapping I used to acquire a bunch of points and then sit back and try to figure out what was going on. This is bad for two reasons: first, you are not using the information you've gathered to decide where to take points, and second, you are not using contextual information to decide when to annotate LAT. As you build a map you may see that there is a clear progression of activation across a region of the heart. If this interpretation "fits" with information around that region then it's probably correct and you don't need more points between these points. If, on the other hand, the data points around

that area are inconsistent with activation spreading uniformly, you may need to investigate a few sites in the middle to confirm whether they truly time "intermediate" between the data points you've acquired thus far.

Some themes

There are two broad types of activation patterns that you'll encounter: focal activation and reentry. In focal activation, isochrones[2] radiate outward from some earliest site (i.e., there is some site from which activation gets later in every direction). This is a pretty easy

---

[2] Lines that connect points with the same activation time.

pattern to identify, although there is one nuance to remember. The isochrones are color-coded and the colors are determined in advance of your map based upon the annotation window you choose. The activation time has an order, with earlier towards the red end of the spectrum and later towards the purple end. Thus when you see colors that "progress" from red (or yellow or green) through successive colors towards purple you easily interpret this as the direction of propagation. It is less intuitive to see that when the colors go from purple to red to yellow that, too, is the direction of propagation. The key is to recognize that timing is relative and that immediately after purple is red. Thus if one doesn't happen to set the left edge of

the annotation window "correctly," earliest may be earlier than red (Figure 10.3).

During reentry there is continuous propagation: the site of "earliest" activation is adjacent to the site of "latest" activation. The mapping system assigns colors to the data points and then it interpolates between them. It interpolates smoothly between data points (i.e., assumes uniform conduction velocity between points). This is pretty straightforward (the only trick is to recognize what's actual data and what's assumption/interpolation) (Figure 10.4).

How does the system interpolate between the latest data point and the earliest? It does exactly what it always does: it draws all the intermediary colors (which in this case is all of them). This is referred to as "reverse" interpolation

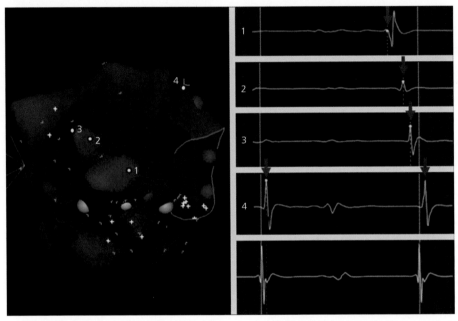

Figure 10.3 Focal activation pattern. Red is not necessarily earliest; activation spreads from earliest (1) to latest (4). Once an electrogram falls to-the-right-of the right edge of the annotation window (4) it is also to-the-right-of the left edge of the window ("early"/red is also immediately *after* purple).

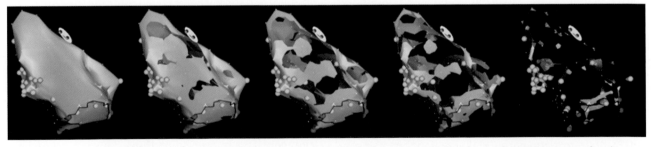

Figure 10.4 Interpolated map vs. actual data. The map on the far left is fully interpolated (there is a color/timing everywhere). Moving from left to right we are decreasing the size of the region we ask the computer to "guess about" (interpolate), revealing how little information we actually have.

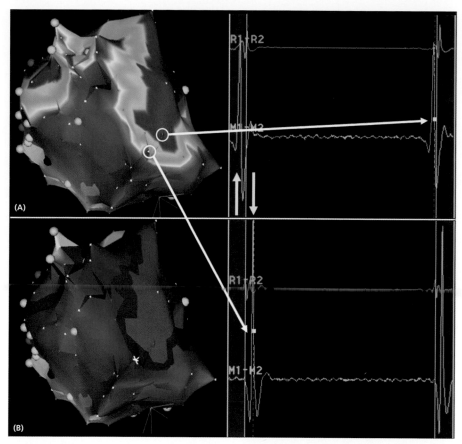

Figure 10.5 Reverse Interpolation. Within the annotation window, red (bottom electrogram) and purple (top electrogram) are at opposite sides of the window (white arrows). In reality, red is immediately *after* purple (yellow arrows). The mapping system interpolates by drawing all the intermediary colors between these two points (just like all the other points). It turns out that *all* the other colors fall between red and purple. The result is referred to as reverse interpolation (top map); it can be distracting to the eye. If you instruct the system to draw a dark red band where "early" meets "late" (bottom map) the colors are less misleading.

(Figure 10.5A). This can be very misleading if you don't recognize what's happening. You can just ignore reverse interpolation when "reading" a map, or some systems allow you to annotate any reverse interpolation points (places where "early meets late") with a dark red band (Figure 10.5B).

Building/refining a map

As you build a map you try to figure out how electricity is spreading and what is driving the rhythm. The first step is to determine the direction(s) of propagation. Follow the progression of colors (remembering not to misinterpret the transition from purple to red). If the activation pattern doesn't make sense, be sure that you are not being misled by interpolated colors. It is common to identify specific areas where more data will help to figure out what's going on. Considering the map in Figure 10.6, you should ask yourself "where is 'blue' coming from?"

You can see that blue leads to purple in three directions. It appears that there is a progression from orange to blue, but on inspection this is entirely interpolated colors, there are no data points.[3] As we acquire more data in this region we see that activation does in fact travel from the orange region to the purple through two areas of scar tissue (gray) (Figure 10.7).

Close inspection reveals that activation actually propagates towards that purple but does not go from purple to red (i.e., it is a dead end). Despite the absence of discernible electrograms in the "scar" region, the contextual information tell us that there must be propagation through the portion of scar adjacent to blue. Rotating the map around allows us to postulate a plausible reentry circuit (Figure 10.8).

---

[3] Data collection points are indicated by small white dots.

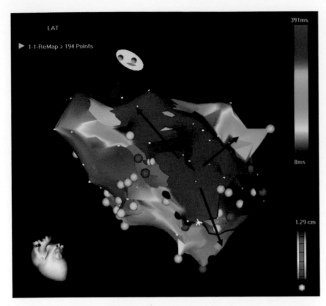

Figure 10.6 Where is "blue" coming from? As you try to interpret a map, it is important to check that you are not basing any of your interpretation on interpolation rather than recorded data.

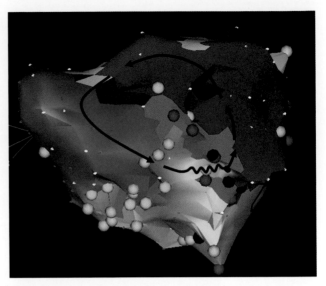

Figure 10.8 Postulated circuit. We see activation through scar tissue on the roof of the left atrium. Where colors are close together there are lots of activation times in a short distance (i.e., slow conduction); this is frequently seen at gaps in scar.

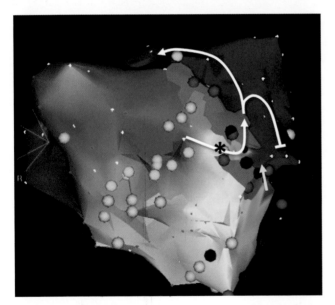

Figure 10.7 Map with more data. The colors on this map look much like the earlier map (which had fewer data points) but in this map the colors in the critical region are due to data points, not interpolation. There is a fractionated signal indicated by the pink dot at * which spans the times between red and green. We do not see any data points within the tissue marked scar (gray) because no electrograms were discernible here. Nonetheless we can deduce that activation traversed through this region, based upon the propagation sequence (blue to purple) emerging from the opposite side of the scar (arrows). The blue color that traverses an apparent gap in the scar (yellow arrow) is actually interpolation (note there are no data points here).

There is a little bit more to note in this map. The rate at which colors change (i.e., the distance between similarly colored points) reveals information about the conduction velocity. The narrow area between scars has very closely spaced isochrones (slow conduction), indicating that nearly half of the cycle length is accounted for by conduction through this narrow isthmus. It turns out this is a common finding. Narrow areas often conduct slowly, and this slow conduction is arrhythmogenic. If we want to ablate so as to transect this circuit we can theoretically do so anywhere, but this narrow isthmus offers the ability to transect the circuit with the shortest possible ablation.

In review, activation mapping requires an electrically stable rhythm: activation must remain the same from beat to beat throughout the duration of map acquisition. The rhythm must also be hemodynamically stable: in other words, the patient must be able to tolerate the rhythm for long enough to create the map. And (obviously) the patient must have the rhythm (they must be inducible or be in tachycardia already).

Substrate mapping

What do we do when the requirements for activation mapping aren't met? There are times when, for any of a number of reasons, we are unable to create an activation map. Under these circumstances, how can we identify the substrate of the patient's rhythm? If there is a structural basis for the arrhythmia, that "structure" is present at all times and can be mapped. In a structural reentrant circuit the potential paths for activation are physically defined, e.g., by scar tissue. Scar can divide the tissue into separate but connected paths for conduction. By mapping the scar tissue (and electrically active tissue) we can identify potential circuits. How do we identify scar? We assume the presence of scar when our catheter is in contact with the tissue but records no (or only far-field) potentials.

The mere presence of a potential circuit is necessary but not sufficient for reentry. The circuit's path length must be greater than the wave length of activation (otherwise "head meets tail" – see Chapter 4). In addition to the presence of scar, areas of slow conduction facilitate reentry by decreasing wave length. Diseased tissue often manifests slow conduction (even during normal rhythm).

When we perform substrate mapping we look for three features: scar tissue (creating non-conducting obstacles), diseased tissue (providing slow conduction), and "channels" (paths through the scar producing circuits). Diseased tissue can be identified by its low voltage (on voltage maps) and slow conduction (on activation maps) (Figure 10.9).

Putting it all together: a case

A final thought about mapping: pay attention to both the "big picture" and the details. In EP we must integrate many streams of data (fluoroscopy, 3D location, electrogram morphology, spatial context, as well as clinical history, e.g., arrhythmia cadence). Often our data are flawed and can be inconsistent. You maximize your chances of success if you capitalize on your tools but understand their limitations. Below is an example that helps to emphasize the need to interpret your map data in the larger context of the information you have about a patient.

Case

A patient presented with drug-resistant atrial tachycardia late after a Mustard repair for transposition of the great vessels. Complicating factors included multiple pulmonary arteriovenous malformations (AVMs) with a room-air saturation of 85% and occlusion of his iliac veins bilaterally. Because of the AVMs we were very hesitant to cross the baffle (to map the systemic atrium) for fear of creating a residual shunt that could exacerbate his baseline hypoxia. Because of the iliac occlusions, we could only approach the atria from the SVC. With that as our context, we made the map shown in Figure 10.10.

Examination of the activation pattern on this map revealed that earliest activation was not adjacent to latest activation, i.e., a focal activation pattern. But there were several hints that the rhythm was not focal.[4] Patients with repaired congenital heart disease have all the components for macro-reentry. They have scar tissue and (frequently) diseased tissue. So while these patients certainly do have focal arrhythmias, macro-reentry is more common. In addition there was the cadence of this patient's rhythm: it was steady and persistent. Automatic or triggered rhythms tend to have a repetitive short bursting behavior rather than very prolonged stable tachycardias.[5] There was one last clue that this might be macro-reentry. Examination of some of the points on the map showed double potentials (not surprising in the context of post-surgical scar). The clue lay in the timing of the potentials (Figure 10.10). The later potential (of the double) was *after* the latest timing in the venous atrial chamber (purple). In addition, the site of the late double potential was near the site of earliest activation. When we considered this in a larger anatomic context (i.e., beyond simply the venous atrial map) the story began to fall together.

We imported the pre-procedural CT image, which indicated that earliest and latest timing in the venous atrium lay at the border between venous and systemic atria (Figure 10.11). This suggested the possibility that there was indeed a macro reentrant circuit involving both chambers. Our map revealed only half of the activation; perhaps a systemic atrial map would reveal a focal activation pattern beginning opposite "purple" and ending opposite "red."

Now what? Again, consider the larger context. Because of the pulmonary AVMs we wanted to avoid crossing the baffle (which would be required to map the systemic atrium). We chose to remain in the venous atrium and performed entrainment.

---

[4] Although micro-reentry remained a reasonable consideration.
[5] Again micro-reentry could explain the cadence.

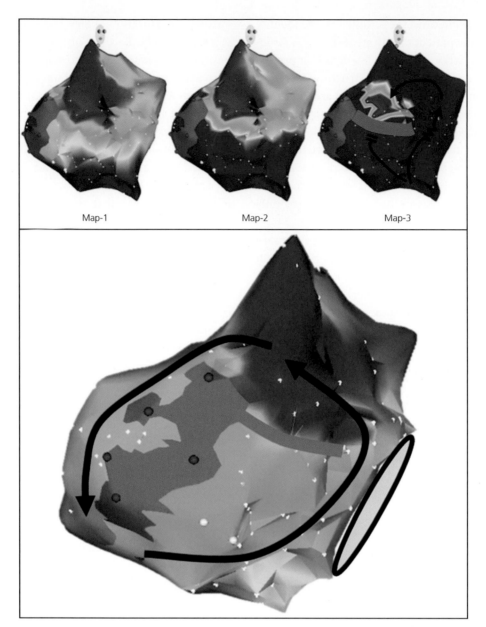

Figure 10.9 Substrate mapping. (Top) *Scar tissue revealed.* In an activation map (performed during CS pacing) the propagation pattern reveals scar. With a quick look at the initial activation map (Map-1) it is not immediately apparent that there is scar in the mid-RA freewall. In Map-1, activation times close to zero are colored red. In Map-2 and Map-3 we have redefined any time less than 120 ms as red. When we manipulate the map colors it becomes more obvious that there is no conduction up the middle of the tissue. (Bottom) *Potential circuit revealed.* This is an activation map but it is acquired during CS pacing (bottom of map). The activation sequence therefore doesn't reveal the circuit (activation is traveling up both sides of the freewall scar (gray). But we have identified a *potential* reentrant circuit (arrows) created by electrically active tissue surrounding the scar. There is an isthmus between the scar and the tricuspid annulus (TA – indicated by the oval) where we subsequently performed a linear ablation.

Where should we entrain? Both the "red" and "purple" sites would be in our putative circuit. We were interested in distinguishing micro-reentry from dual-chamber macro-reentry. The "red" site was in both putative circuits while the "purple" site was only in the macro-reentrant circuit. Entrainment from the "purple" site was consistent with dual-chamber macro-reentry. The "red" site was the entry site into the venous atrium (Figure 10.10). Ablation at this site terminated tachycardia, which was then no longer inducible.

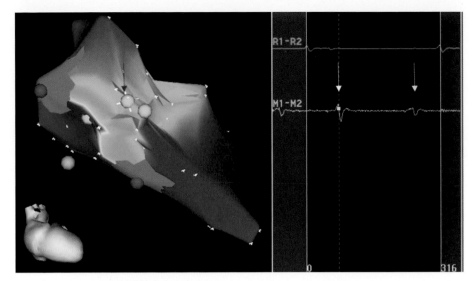

Figure 10.10 Activation map in a patient with a Mustard repair. The area of earliest activation (red) is not adjacent to the area of latest activation (purple). This seems to indicate a focal tachycardia (with reentry there is continuous conduction, so early activation *has to be adjacent to* late activation). Note that purple on this map is at 125 ms although the tachycardia cycle length is 316 ms. In a focal rhythm there is no reason that the tachycardia cycle length must equal the total conduction time (in reentry they must be equal). Note, however, that there is a double potential (red arrow). The local activation time (earlier deflection – white arrow) is 76 ms; the later potential (yellow arrow) is at 265 ms, which is *later than* the latest time in the map (purple is 125 ms). This definitively indicates that we have not yet mapped all of activation – in fact we are missing more than half of the tachycardia cycle length.

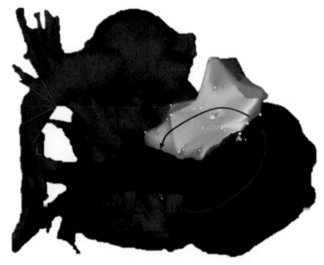

Figure 10.11 Venous and systemic atria. When we combine the CT image of this patient's heart with the activation map of the venous atrium, we see that both "red" and "purple" are adjacent to the systemic chamber. This, plus the entrainment mapping, suggests a bi-atrial circuit (arrows).

Summary

- Activation mapping: requires a physically and electrically stable reference.
- Set the annotation window to the tachycardia cycle length (TCL). Set the window: left edge at 0 ms, right edge at TCL (easier to detect changes in cycle length).
- Colors are relative: don't be fooled into thinking red = earliest.
- Double potentials: indicate local block. In the presence of linear block (line of double potentials) pay attention to which direction is "early" and which is "late," and annotate double potentials accordingly (do the same with fractionated signals).
- Be cognizant of what colors are due to interpolation vs. data.
- Focal activation: early is not (necessarily) adjacent to late (be aware that purple can precede red).
- Reentrant activation: early meets late; all activation times are accounted for; beware of reverse interpolation.
- Substrate mapping: look for anatomically defined potential circuits: scar, channels, and diseased tissue (low amplitude, slow conduction).

Appendix: What we measure when we record an electrogram

In this section we discuss the relationship between electric current (the stuff that happens in the heart) and the electric field that it produces (the stuff we are able to record). Understanding this relationship is critical to effectively practice clinical EP. Many mistakes arise from a failure to appreciate that electrograms are *not* a direct measure of cardiac propagation. By understanding what we are measuring, how it is influenced by the electrodes we use, and the spatial relationship between those electrodes and the heart, we minimize the likelihood that we will misinterpret our recordings.

This review may delve more deeply into the underlying math than some readers would prefer. There are equations to make the story complete for those who are interested; but it is not critical that you follow along with the math. For those *not* mathematically inclined, I highly recommend that you read this anyway. You can put your fingers in your ears during the equations and still grasp the important principles.

Electricity and the electric field

Atoms are made up of a variety of components. Two of the most important are *electrons* and *protons*, which carry equal and opposite electric charges. What exactly is electric charge, and why do electrons and protons have it? … No one knows. What we do know is that electrons and protons are attracted to each other and repel their own kind. This property is, in fact, what it means to have electric charge. We also know from experiments that all electrons carry exactly the same charge, which by convention is defined to be of a negative sign. Protons are found to have a charge of the same magnitude as the electron, but of the opposite (positive) sign.

Isolated atoms have equal numbers of protons and electrons and are therefore electrically neutral. Some combinations of atoms may share their electrons in a way that binds them together as molecules. Collections of metal atoms are able to share electrons in a way that allows them to move freely from one atom to the next, even though the net balance of positive and negative charges remains unchanged. Electrons in metals can thus flow in a steady stream as an *electric current*. Salts dissolved in water are also able to support electric currents because the salt molecules, which are electrically neutral when dry, break up in solution into positively charged and negatively charged *ions* that are able to move independently of each other.

Although electrons are able to move about freely in a *conductor* such as a metal, they will only move in a given direction, as an electric current, if there is some force driving them along. This force arises from the *electric field*, a concept developed by Michael Faraday that helps us understand how two charged bodies can push or pull on each other without actually touching. The way to think of an electric field is to realize that a charged body is more than simply a mass located somewhere in space. In addition, the charge on the body changes the property of space itself by setting up an electric field that stretches all the way out to infinity. The strength, E, of this field falls off with the square of the distance away from the body, eventually becoming negligible when far enough away. E is also proportional to the charge, q, on the body (i.e., on the number of unbalanced electrons or protons it contains). We can thus say that

$$E = \frac{\varepsilon_0 q}{r^2} \tag{1}$$

Understanding Clinical Cardiac Electrophysiology: A Conceptually Guided Approach, First Edition. Peter Spector.
© 2016 John Wiley & Sons, Inc. Published 2016 by John Wiley & Sons, Inc.
Companion website: www.wiley.com/go/spector/cardiac_electrophysiology

where ε_0 is a constant of proportionality[1] known as the *permittivity* of the material comprising the region of space in which the charges are located. Free space has a particular value for ε_0, which is different from other materials such as water, air, etc.

It is worth pointing out that the inverse square law for E actually makes intuitive sense if one thinks of the strength of the field as reflecting the rate at which some material emanates uniformly out in all directions from a charged body. By analogy, imagine a spherical rubber balloon that is inflating outward from a central point. As the radius, r, of the balloon increases, its surface area increases as $4\pi r^2$. The amount of rubber making up the wall of the balloon isn't changing (as you blow it up/increase r) that rubber is simply spread more thinly over the increased surface area of the balloon. The area increases faster than the radius increases; area is increasing in two dimensions whereas the radius is only increasing in one. So the amount of rubber at any given spot on the balloon is *decreasing* faster than r is increasing (i.e., it decreases as $1/r^2$).

Equation 1 tells us how big the electric field is at any point in space, but there is more to it than just its magnitude. The electric field at any point also has a *direction* defined by the fact that it decreases in magnitude at the greatest rate as one moves directly away from the charge. Now we need to think of r in Eq. 1 as a radius *vector*, essentially an arrow pointing from the charge to a particular point in space. E itself is then also a vector, written $\vec{E}$, having the same direction as the radius vector but with magnitude given by Eq. 1. Rewriting Eq. 1 as a *vector equation* gives

$$\vec{E} = \frac{\varepsilon_0 q}{r^2}\hat{r} \qquad (2)$$

where $\hat{r}$ is the so-called *unit radius vector* that points away from the charge and has a magnitude of 1. Vector equations must not only have the same magnitude on both sides, they must also point in the same direction.

---

[1] For those of you who recoil at all things math, ε_0 is a number (that doesn't change for any given medium) which can be larger or smaller depending upon how easily space filled with that medium is altered by charge.

Coulomb's law

When a charged body finds itself bathed in the electric field of another charged body, the first particle experiences a force proportional both to its own charge and to the strength of the local electric field. The force is directed toward the other particle if the two particles have opposite charge and away from it if their charges are the same. Force, like the electric field, is thus also a vector – $\vec{F}$. If the charges on the first and second bodies are q_1 and q_2, respectively, then

$$\begin{aligned} \vec{F} &= \vec{E}q_2 \\ &= \frac{\varepsilon_0 q_1 q_2}{r^2}\hat{r} \end{aligned} \qquad (3)$$

Equation 3 is known as *Coulomb's law* after the scientist who discovered it experimentally. Interestingly, Coulomb's law has exactly the same mathematical form as Newton's law of gravity, except that the force in Coulomb's law can be either positive or negative depending on whether the charges on the bodies in question are the same or opposite.

In real-world applications, one is rarely faced with a situation as simple as only two point charges. Usually, there are many charges situated at various locations around the position of interest, so calculating the total force on a test charge at a given point is not as simple as using Eq. 3. Fortunately, the impact of various charges on the electric field at any point in space simply adds together, a principle known as *superposition*. It is important to remember, though, that these individual fields add like vectors. So, for example, if two identical charges are located at equal distances away from a particular point in space but in precisely opposite directions, their resultant field at that point is zero regardless of how big the individual field magnitudes might be. Thus, the force on a test charge q is given by the vector sum

$$\begin{aligned} \vec{F} &= \sum_i \vec{E}_i q \\ &= q\sum_i \frac{\varepsilon_0 q_i}{r_i^2}\hat{r}_i \end{aligned} \qquad (4)$$

The electric potential field

So far, we have been considering interactions between charges that are fixed in space. Coulomb's law provides the forces such charges exert on each other, but there are no consequences to these forces unless the charges are able to move, so now let us suppose that movement is possible. In particular, imagine that a fixed charge q_1 exerts a repulsive force on a second charge q_2 located a distance r away, and that this second charge is free to move in whatever direction it is pushed. Now the electric field generated by q_1 is able to do *work* on q_2 by pushing it away.

Recall that the work done on a body is defined as the product of the distance moved by the body and the force applied in the direction of movement. In vector terms, this is given by the *dot product* of the force vector and the displacement vector integrated over the total path that the body moves. In the case of one charge moving away from another, the force and displacement vectors are always co-linear, so the total work, W, done on q_2 when it moves away from q_1 by a certain distance, say out to r_2, is given by the integral

$$W = \int_{r_1}^{r_2} \frac{\varepsilon_0 q_1 q_2}{r^2} \, dr$$

$$= -\varepsilon_0 q_1 q_2 \left[\frac{1}{r} \right]_r^{r_2} \qquad (5)$$

$$= \varepsilon_0 q_1 q_2 \frac{r_2 - r}{r r_2}$$

We have used only the magnitude part of Eq. 3 in Eq. 5 because the movement of charge q_2 is always in the direction of the electric field generated by charge q_1.

Now assume that charge q_2 is allowed to move off infinitely far away from q_1, which it will do if nothing stops it. This means that r_2 tends to infinity, causing $(r_2 - r)$ in the numerator of Eq. 5 to become simply r_2. This cancels with the r_2 in the denominator so that Eq. 5 becomes simply

$$W = \frac{e_0 q_1 q_2}{r}$$

$$= \frac{E q_1}{r} \qquad (6)$$

In other words, the amount of work that the electric field from a point charge can potentially do by pushing a second test charge off to infinity is inversely proportional to the distance, r, between the two charges. If we let q_1 be unity, then W is defined to be the *electric potential*, Φ, at the point in space where the test charge is located. That is,

$$\Phi = \frac{E}{r} \qquad (7)$$

Note that E in Eq. 7 is just the magnitude of the electric field because the direction of the field is irrelevant for calculating Φ. Φ has a definite value at every point in space (i.e., it is a field). Unlike the electric field, however, Φ is a *scalar field*, having magnitude but no direction.[2]

Ohm's law

When a charge is moved between two points having potentials Φ_1 and Φ_2, respectively, by the force of an electric field, it must be pushed along against the *resistance* offered by the physical presence of the other matter it meets between the two points. If the charge moves at a constant velocity then there is no change in its kinetic energy as it makes this journey, so the energy that it loses is merely the potential energy difference, $\Delta\Phi$, between the two points, which is equal to $\Phi_1 - \Phi_2$. This lost potential energy is converted to an equivalent amount of heat energy as a result of the path having a finite resistance to movement of the charge. If many charges are moved in a steady stream from Φ_1 to Φ_2 then the total work done is proportional to the number of charges. The flow of charge between two points of different potential is thus precisely analogous to the flow of water through a narrow hose.

The situation just described can be expressed in mathematical terms as follows. First, $\Delta\Phi$ is defined as the *voltage*, V, between the two points of different electric potential, and is analogous to the pressure that drives water through a hose. Next, the number of charge carriers per second that move past a given point between Φ_1 and Φ_2 is called the *current*, I, and is analogous to the volume of water flow through a hose. Finally, just as a hose offers a resistance to the flow of water, so does a conducting pathway offer a resistance, R, to the flow of electric current. The mathematical relationship describing the relationship between voltage, current and resistance is known as *Ohm's law*, written as

$$V = IR \qquad (8)$$

The way that the voltage between two points is measured is also described by Ohm's law. The essence

---

[2] A field made up of values that have magnitude but no direction is called a *scalar field*; one made up of values that have both magnitude and direction is called a *vector field*.

of the approach is to connect an additional conducting pathway between the two points, so that charge carriers now have two parallel pathways along which they can make the journey. Of crucial importance, the resistance, R_2, of this second pathway must be known, and also must be much greater than that of the original pathway so that only a very small amount of the charge carriers choose this second (measuring) pathway. If the measuring pathway's resistance is very high, flow through it will be small enough that it will not have a significant effect on the current flow through the original pathway. The tiny current flow along the second pathway is then measured and used in Eq. 8 with R replaced by the known value R_2 to provide V.

Ohm's law is usually written as shown in Eq. 8, because this is appropriate for describing the flow of electricity around an entire electric *circuit*. Ohm's law can also be written in local form, however, so that it applies to an infinitesimally small region of space. Here, instead of talking about a flow of current from one point to another, we refer to *current density*, j, which is simply the current per unit cross-sectional area that flows past a particular point of interest. To convert between these two representations of current, we divide I by the area, A, across which it flows. That is,

$$j = I/A \tag{9}$$

Note that the current at a point in space flows in a particular direction, as opposed to the current around a circuit which does not have a single direction associated with it because the direction of the circuit has to change in order to make a closed loop. j is thus the magnitude of a vector quantity.

The local equivalent of R in Eq. 8 is called *resistivity*, ρ, and it is equal to the resistance of a segment of the material making up the conducting pathway that has unit cross-sectional area and unit length. The resistivity of a segment *increases* as its length, l, increases, but *decreases* as its area, A, increases; a larger area means more parallel pathways for the current to flow through. The relationship between ρ and R is therefore

$$\rho = RA/l \tag{10}$$

Finally, the local equivalent of the voltage drop, V, from Eq. 8 is the *voltage per unit distance* in the direction of current flow; this is none other than the strength of the electric field at the point of interest. That is,

$$E = V/l \tag{11}$$

The local form of Ohm's law is thus the vector equation

$$\vec{E} = \vec{j}\rho \tag{12}$$

assuming that the resistivity of the material involved is isotropic so that ρ is a scalar. Equation 12 can be verified by substituting Eqs. 9–11 into Eq. 12 to obtain Eq. 8.

As a special case of Eq. 12, consider an isolated point source of current having intensity I, such as might describe a tiny battery bathed in a uniform conducting medium extending out to infinity in all directions. Because of the symmetry of the situation, the flow of charge produced by this battery moves out uniformly in all directions, driven by an electric field that always points away from the battery and that falls off in strength as the square of the distance away. The current density and the electric field strength at any point in the medium are thus both functions only of radial distance, r, from the battery. Since electric charge is conserved, the current can be thought of as a fixed number of moving charges proportional to I that are uniformly spread out over a sphere of area $4\pi r^2$, making the strength of the current density and the electric field at any point proportional to $I/4\pi r^2$. That is, from Eq. 12,

$$\begin{aligned} j(r) &= E(r)/\rho \\ &= I/4\pi r^2 \end{aligned} \tag{13}$$

Recording the intracardiac electrogram

What we have just described is a basic model of what happens when the tip of a recording electrode inside the beating heart measures the electrical activity of a depolarizing heart cell. The uniform conducting medium in this case is the blood that bathes the electrode tip and connects it electrically to the heart tissue. When a heart cell located a distance r from the electrode tip becomes electrically excited, a small amount of current flows between the inside and the outside of the cell. This creates an electrical disturbance in the nearby blood where local charge carriers move in an attempt to counteract the changing electric field created by the movement of charge that occurred in the cell. In other words, a current source arises in the blood adjacent to the cell with a strength essentially proportional to the rate of depolarization of the cell. The electric field strength at a distance r from the cell is thus, by Eq. 13, equal to $I\rho/4\pi r^2$. The potential measured by an electrode at a distance r due to this one depolarizing cell, in analogy with Eq. 7, is therefore $j\rho/4\pi r$.

Of course, at any instant in time there are, in general, many cells in the process of depolarizing simultaneously, each making a contribution to the total potential, Φ, recorded by the electrode. It is Φ, as a function of time, that constitutes the intracardiac electrogram. To express Φ mathematically for a sheet of excitable tissue, we define the position of the electrode tip to be (x_e, y_e, z_e) with respect to some set of Cartesian coordinates. The current density at the tissue surface then becomes a continuous function of these coordinates. The combined contributions to Φ from this continuous current density are then given by the integral

$$\Phi\left(x_e, y_e, z_e\right) = \frac{\rho}{4\pi} \iiint_{x\,y\,z} \frac{j\left(x, y, z\right)}{\sqrt{\left(x-x_e\right)^2 + \left(y-y_e\right)^2 + \left(z-z_e\right)^2}} \, dz\,dy\,dx$$

(14)

What we have just described is a simple model of Φ that ignores many of the details of reality. For example, cardiac tissue has a finite thickness, so some of the depolarizing cells that contribute to Φ are surrounded by other cells rather than blood. Also, the flow of current associated with depolarizing cells is more complicated than simple movement of ions between the exterior and interior of each cell; balancing currents also exist between adjacent cells and in a lateral direction exterior to cell–cell junctions. Nevertheless, Eq. 13 captures the dominant processes leading to the generation of Φ, and therefore produces realistic electrogram morphologies when applied to models of the two-dimensional propagation of electrical excitation in the heart. The formula also captures the relationship between the tissue's electrical activity and the electrode's recording sufficiently to allow an intuitive feel for how electrode location and size impact electrogram recordings.

Afterword: Your heart is a computer: from army ants to atrial fibrillation

The normal heartbeat is a wonder of communication and coordination between millions of individual cells. Each cell is capable of pulsating on its own; left to their own devices the cells of the heart would constitute nothing but a quivering mass of tissue serving no useful purpose. However, by passing just the right amount of electrical excitation from cell to cell, in exactly the right sequence, the entire population is able to produce the heartbeat, the singular event required for pumping blood around the body.

The coordinated activity of myriad potentially independent agents toward a common higher purpose, one that is beyond the capabilities of any of the agents alone, is the hallmark of any useful system. Indeed, the biosphere is essentially a collection of such systems manifest at all conceivable scales of length and time. An archetypical example is a colony of army ants, a system capable of building huge intricate structures, surviving climatic hardship, and spawning copies of itself, all despite the very limited skill sets of its individual agents (the ants). Furthermore, there is no boss ant telling the other ants what to do. The ant colony achieves its remarkable global feats simply by having each ant follow a simple set of rules that dictate its actions relative to the other ants and to the environment in which it finds itself. The result is that although each ant's activities might impinge directly only on those ants in its immediate vicinity, the cooperative nature of these activities causes their effects to be amplified up to the level of the entire system.

The coordinated activity of relatively simple agents also characterizes useful man-made systems, from the humblest child's toy up to a nuclear submarine, but is perhaps no better exemplified than in the digital computer. Here, an enormous collection of interconnected elements, each of which is capable only of implementing a small number of Boolean logic operations, is able to collectively implement arbitrarily complex sets of instructions. These instructions (the computer program) define the simple rules by which each logic element is to operate, and in which order. In this sense, the digital computer and the ant colony have strong formal similarities, even though their respective agents are very different. Also, in the case of the ant colony, the software has been selected by evolution rather than by a scientist's design. Nevertheless, what eventually emanates from both systems is the consequence of a large number of simple rules having been followed in the correct order and at the correct time. In other words, both the computer and the ant colony perform calculations.

The above analogy extends immediately to the heart. Although an individual heart cell is miraculously complex in all its details, its behavior in essence is very simple; either it remains quiescent, or it becomes electrically excited and puts its contractile machinery into operation for a brief period of time. When the heart is working properly, this "decision" is made on the basis of interactions with adjacent heart cells. A normal contraction of the entire heart requires this decision to be made by all the heart cells in precisely the correct order and at precisely the right time, just like the calculations in a computer. Of course, digital computers are not exactly like the heart in this regard because a single wrong step in one of the logic operations in a computer is likely to yield an erroneous calculation, whereas the heart can do just fine with a few cells that do not work properly. This difference, however, is just an issue with current computer architectures which employ serial operations; future computer designs may well make use

Understanding Clinical Cardiac Electrophysiology: A Conceptually Guided Approach, First Edition. Peter Spector.
© 2016 John Wiley & Sons, Inc. Published 2016 by John Wiley & Sons, Inc.
Companion website: www.wiley.com/go/spector/cardiac_electrophysiology

of parallel processing and be robust to a certain degree of hardware failure. The point is that the heart does a calculation that tells it exactly how to behave.

Because each of the millions of individual cells in the heart can potentially become activated in any order, and at any point in time, there is a virtually unlimited number of possible software programs that the heart computer can run. The normal program, the one that results in the normal heartbeat, is actually pretty boring because it produces a simple wave of excitation that sweeps over the heart in the same way beat after beat. Much more interesting calculations can be made by the heart (based upon the cell properties, tissue architecture, and "initial conditions") such that cell excitation proceeds in any number of patterns, some quite disorganized or continuously varying. Unfortunately, exciting though this might be from a computational perspective, from the point of view of sustaining life the result can be catastrophic. In fact, one of the most common forms of cardiac arrhythmia, atrial fibrillation, is precisely what happens when an interesting calculation of this nature is made by the atrial chambers of the heart.

The heart really is a computer. Understanding how the heart works normally, and what happens when it goes wrong, thus requires that we understand the calculations that it makes.

Burton Sobel, Jason Bates,
and Peter Spector

Suggested reading

Bers, D. *Excitation Contraction Coupling and Cardiac Contractile Force*, 2nd edition. Kluwer Academic Publishers, 2001.

Flake, G. W. *The Computational Beauty of Nature*. MIT Press, 1998.

Jalife, J., Delmar, M., Anumonwo, J., Berenfeld, O., and Kalifa, J. *Basic Cardiac Electrophysiology for the Clinician*, 2nd edition. John Wiley & Sons, Inc., 2009.

Mitchell, M. *Complexity: A Guided Tour*. Oxford University Press, 2011.

Surawicz, B. *Electrophysiologic Basis of ECG and Cardiac Arrhythmias*. Williams & Wilkins, 1995.

Wit, A. L., and Janse, M. J. *The Ventricular Arrhythmias of Ischemia and Infarction: Electrophysiological Mechanisms*. Futura Publishing Company, 1993.

Index

Page numbers in *italics* refer to figures

Understanding Clinical Cardiac Electrophysiology: A Conceptually Guided Approach, First Edition. Peter Spector.
© 2016 John Wiley & Sons, Inc. Published 2016 by John Wiley & Sons, Inc.
Companion website: www.wiley.com/go/spector/cardiac_electrophysiology